MAIDEN.

A MOTHER'S GUIDE TO PUBERTY AND MENARCHE AS A SACRED RITE OF PASSAGE

DONNA RAYMOND

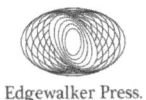

Edgewalker Press.

Maiden. A Mother's Guide To Puberty And Menarche As A Sacred Rite Of Passage

Published by Edgewalker Press 2021

First Edition 2021

Copyright © 2021 Donna Raymond, Wise Wombman

All rights reserved. No part of this publication may be reproduced, stored in a retrieval system, or transmitted in any form or by any means, electronic, mechanical, photocopying, recording or otherwise, without the prior written permission from both the copyright owner and publisher.

Disclaimer

All the information, techniques, skills and concepts contained within this publication are of the nature of general comment only and are not in any way recommended as individual advice. The intent is to offer a variety of information to provide a wider range of choices now and in the future, recognising that we all have widely diverse circumstances and viewpoints. Should any reader choose to make use of the information contained herein, this is their decision and the author and publishers do not assume any responsibilities whatsoever under any condition or circumstances.

Cover design: Donna Raymond

Editing: Donna Hakanson

Printing: Eureka Printing PTY LTD

ISBN: 978-0-6450968-1-1

Visit: www.wisewombman.com

MAIDEN.

*For our daughters
Across all timelines past, present and future!*

May our girls be welcomed into womanhood in a way that is honouring and fosters deep connection to their blood, body and sensual power as feminine beings.

*May they connect with the Mother Earth and her innate primal and cyclic wisdom.
May they connect with their womb, heart and throat and feel free to sing in celebration, for their blood is Sacred.*

---

*To my kind, intelligent and beautiful daughters:
Auraura, Maia and Lucah…
May your wombs be blessed and may you pass this wisdom on when you are called.*

Menarche

The Ancient red thread
Stitches stories to my womb
Mother, mother
I am in full bloom.
With tender petals, I unfurl
Touching the surface of a new world
Gently embracing the unknown
I am no longer a little girl.
From child to woman
I now flow
The Great Mysteries revealed
I'm ready to let go.
Grandmother moon whispers her secrets
Keeper of seasons and cycles
I remember.

The portal opens.
I take a step forward.
I am here now
I am a Maiden

In this primal wilderness
The Sacred threads unravel

prayers of bleeding women's wisdom
Weaving language around my crimson
The Womb a sacred site of blood rites
And I surrender to the flow

From womb to tomb
I stand initiated

Shedding the skin of who I was
Discovering the woman I am now
And am now becoming

I am a Maiden

© copyright Donna Raymond 2021

CONTENTS

Foreword   13
Endorsements   15
Acknowledgments   17
Preface   23
Introduction   27

1. PREPARING FOR WOMANHOOD   31
2. PUBERTY AS AN INITIATION   37
   Puberty Brain   39
   Hormones   40
   Menarche: A Rite Of Passage   42
   The Revival Of Ceremony As A Spiritual Practice   44
   Overcoming Cultural Shame + Stigma   45
3. REPRODUCTIVE / SEXUAL HEALTH AND WELLBEING   49
   The Biology of the Menstrual Cycle   51
   How Stress Affects the Menstrual Cycle   53
   Late and Abnormal Cycle   54
   Cycle Mapping   56
   Education Leads To Empowerment   59
   Books To Educate And Inspire   62
   Menstruation Books: 62
   Educational Websites   63
   Menstrual Apps for electronic devices   64
4. MAIDEN/MENARCHE CELEBRATION CEREMONY   65
   Asking Permission   65
   The Power Of Ritual   67

Setting The Space 68
What is An Altar? 69
How To Create Your Menarche Altar 70

5. MENARCHE RITUAL IDEAS 73
Blessing + Gift 73
Ritual Menstrual Candle 74
How To Create Your Rolled Candle 75
Time Capsule 77
Spiral Labyrinth 78
Shared Artwork 79
Guide Stones 79
Flower Crowns 81
Weaving the Womb Web- The Red Thread 81
Red Stains and Offerings 82
Taking Advantage Of Technology 83
Photo Shoot. 84
Healing Your Own Maiden 84
Menstrual Basket 86
Honouring Neurodiversity 88

Maiden Ceremony Photos 91

6. HOW TO CREATE YOUR CEREMONY TEMPLATE 99
Opening- 99
Welcome- 101
Introduction- 101
Transition- 102
Ritual or Activity- 102
Close- 103
Piecing It All together 103
Potent Transmissions 103

7. MENSTRUAL MAJICK AND THE CEREMONY OF BLEEDING 107
Mystical Wombspace 107
Womb Wisdom 108

Womb Blood is Sacred	109
Collecting Womb Blood	112
Majickal Moon Cycles	112
Blood Rituals For Teens	114
Womb Steaming	116
The Red Tent Movement.	118
Final Words Of Wisdom	121
Auraura's Experience- In Her Words	125
Words from NanaH	129
Find A Women's Circle	133
About the Author	141
Wise Wombman Wisdom School	143
Notes…	145

FOREWORD

Welcome!

I am so glad you found this book. I know you're going to find it such a helpful and inspiring resource.

Being a mama is beautiful but tough work. You want to get it right. But what is right? Often all you know is that you want it to be different…better…more meaningful…than how it was for you. This is our driving force for our children. This book is such a gift if you are approaching your daughter's first bleeding looking for guidance on what to do and how to prepare. It provides wisdom and support on every level: emotional, practical and ceremonial, and the knowledge that you…and your precious daughter are not alone in this momentous transition. Other mothers and daughters have walked this path before you. Here is some of their wisdom.

I love the fact that the focus is put on preparing our daughters gradually as they grow up, as this is instinctively the path I took myself. Learning about our own menstrual cycles and sharing this knowledge with our daughters is the best initiation we can give them – whatever their age - there is no such thing as "too early" or "too late". Doing this we are breaking the silence of previous generations and cultural norms through our living practice.

As a mother of two girls of this age, and an author who has written about menstruation and ritual for well over a decade, I found Maiden both fresh and wise. But even more importantly I felt safe and held reading it. As a neurodivergent mother to a neurodivergent daughter I am particularly grateful to Donna for naming and exploring approaches for our community. The biggest take away that I hope you get from this book is that supporting our menstrual selves is shared and ongoing work. And celebrating our daughters must always put their unique needs front and center.

Lucy H. Pearce, author of *Moon Time; Reaching for the Moon; Medicine Woman; Burning Woman*, founder *Womancraft Publishing*.

ENDORSEMENTS

"This book is a practical guide book for mothers about menarche, a girl's first period. It has everything a mother needs to know to welcome her daughter to a positive menstrual cycle experience, and to heal her own past wounds of menstrual shame in the process. This book helps mothers on:

How to nurture our daughters into being sovereign women. How to help our daughters see the cultural game of sexualisation of maidenhood so they can choose a different path where they are honoured as they are rather than measured by their desirability physically. How to do ceremony to welcome girls to womanhood… and so much more"

Jane Hardwicke Collings, Founder of The School of Shamanic Womancraft

"**MAIDEN** is an essential offering that is needed not only in our community of women, but as an essential element for the evolving human species as we come back into balance with nature, with each other, indeed with all Life.

As women and their daughters reclaim their sacred rites of passage, a guidebook and catalysis to our intrinsic deeper knowing of the wisdom of our bodies is a much welcomed gift. This is love letter written from wise experience and remembrance. Be sure to add it to your collection, for yourself and future generations."

Sarah Drew-author of GAIA CODEX: *A Novel and Ancient Wisdom Text Revealed*

ACKNOWLEDGMENTS

Firstly I would like to acknowledge the traditional custodians of the land, songlines and dreaming tracks, the Djabugay and Bulwai Bama of Kuranda, North Queensland, Australia. This country speaks to me, and I am so blessed to live on this ancient land and be continuously inspired by the surrounding Rainforest and all the mythical stories that are anchored into the landscape. I would also like to acknowledge my ancestors and your ancestors, especially the maternal line and all women who have walked before us, across all dimensions and timelines.

It is important and respectful to acknowledge the women who have been silenced, cast aside and riddled with shame because of their menstrual blood. I can only imagine what that would feel like and I feel that it is important to use my privilege to speak up for those whose voices are and were not heard. We can do better sister, and we will, we are!

I would like to take a moment to acknowledge all of the women on the forefront of this movement, sharing their wisdom and educating other women, mothers and young girls. To my peers, the dedication and work you have put in over decades has paved the way for a new generation of women to have access to this wisdom that is accessible and relatable. I honour your courage for leading and offering your gifts to the world when it may not have been ready to receive them fully. They and you do not go unnoticed. Thank you, I appreciate you!

Heather, you have been an incredible Mother and although we clashed in many ways during my very ordinary initiation into womanhood, I am so grateful for the way that you raised me and encouraged me to dream big and ask questions. Thank you for teaching me how to think outside the box, for challenging me to grow and always having my back, whilst giving me the blunt Sagittarian truth when I don't want it, but need to hear it. I am so grateful for your generosity in financially backing my wild business education endeavours and creativity. I don't know how to repay you so I'll keep creating and serving so that your legacy lives on through me, and your grandchildren. I'm also grateful that you kinda go along with my weird ideas and by now know to trust me when I tell you what we're doing. You are like the ultimate ride or die partner, only now your hair is long and white and I'm taller than you, so you're more like my witchy sidekick!

One of the most beautiful things I have witnessed is your bond and connection with my children, no words will ever suffice in explaining how that reaches my heart, to see you mothering them and loving them as you do. Watching Auraura receive her menarche gift from you, with the little jelly bean centre was simply precious and still makes me tear up. A treasured memory for sure! Through your blood I am here. And so are these words. I am so blessed to be your daughter and to learn how to be an incredible Mother, and someday Maga/Crone from you. I love you.

To my beautiful friend Donni, thank you for being so generous with your time and eyesight. HA! I would often look forward to opening the edited manuscript to see the yellow highlighted text jump out at me and of course, read your thoughtful commentary. I appreciate you and you help with making sure this manuscript could sing on it's own.

Nainiouman Coya Coya, my dear and wise sister, thank you for investing in the creation of this book and the stoking of the fire that has now birthed the Edgewalker Press publishing house. Thank you for seeing the vision of legacy and supporting my dreaming. I love you and am forever grateful for our kinship. You have taught me so much about Lore over the years and I am blessed when the wind and Spirit carries you to my door for a yarn, a laugh and of course a cuppa. You are always welcome in my home tidda!

Chanel, your friendship and enthusiasm to continually collaborate on many creative projects together are so deeply treasured and valued. You have been there for me in many ways during pivotal moments of growth in my life and business. I love you! I love that we are a dream team of creativity! You captured the essence of the Menarche ceremony so beautifully and I love that we get to share these incredible photographs with the world! They say images speak more than a thousand words, and so you my dear Chaneli, have the ability to transcend all barriers of language, translating ephemeral moments that speak to the Soul directly. Just… fabulous daahhling!!!

I would like to acknowledge my sister Joanne, Toddi, Meagan and Sue for helping to create such a memorable ceremony for Auraura, your open sharing helped my daughter to feel seen and connected to something bigger than herself. To Madi, thankyou for the way you tend to the Earth with such devotion and offering such beautiful blooms of colour and fragrance, your garden always lifts my Spirit. Jolene, your yoni cakes were a hit and I am so grateful for your generosity in providing such novelty treats!

To all of the mothers I had conversations with over the years, to the ones who asked me hundreds of questions that stimulated the focus on what to write about, and to the mothers who shared their personal wisdom of experience, I honour all of your contributions to make this book possible, your legacy lives through these words too.

To all of the incredible humans who pledged towards the Kickstarter campaign to get the first edition printed!

The Creative Fund by BackerKit, Jess Russell, Michelle Coppard, Amelia McCutcheon, Ratsimbazafy Stephanie, Helen French, Debbie savage, Chanel Baran, Erika, Zara Walton, Gina Martin, Amy Simpkins, Sergey Kochergan, Kylie Arantzz, Catherine Taylor, Nicola Bryars-Parker, Anne-Marie Owen, Tessa Merten, Libby Penning, Chira Heally, Joyelle Petersen, Emilie Alciato, Sabrina Elmaliah, Katy Maya, Karina Ladet, Shantelle Clarke, Janja, Jess, Jessie Vardakis, Marissa Reid, Donni Didit, Jessy Lynch, Narelle Dichiera, Davini, Erin Black, Nikki Sporri, Kylie Parker, Femke Lemberg, Sarah Slater, Emma Bruce, Maria

Gillies, Georgina Cox, Niomi Reardon, Sabrina Drury, Jaye Harris, Marie Zonruiter, Janine Le Roux, Bek Grundy, Karrie Da Barri Jennings, Emma Exum, Nicole, Lucy, Sarah Drew, Shelly Langford, Emily Welham, Ciara Bridgland, Amy Hatlan, Rhianna, Lunna Valerie Pergay, Kiera, Tania, Antje, Ashlee Benson, Lila Lisa, Crystal-jade Thrives, Jacqueline Rolandelli, Mumma Mae, Beth Norwood, Amber Katri, Freedom Lē Burns, Emma, Kathy Popplewell, Jillian Zamora, Ann-Marie Donnelly, Sophie Jacob McGrath, Nickie Comley, Ember Spring Jaiah, SEGURA, MaddieL Sophie Wicksteed, Melissa, Rochelle, Teala Regan, Jodie Yamada-Colwell, Relle, Megan Denning, Sandra Bacchi, Irena Deacon, Meagan Mitchelson, Tracey, Kerri, Nálii Krééture, Sue Higgins, Gabi, Jenny Lane, Kim Darby, Sara, Erin Reece, Snow Family, Donna Pickford, Dania, Nathacha Subero, Rebecca Reid, Tonielle Christensen, Emily, Kyla, Deirdre Gleeson, Veela Jeweline, Tom O'Connor, Jenine Batless, Bianca Haakman, Zara, Freya Gould, Rebecca Guidera, Meleuka, Wantungaa Wantungaa, Sharee Carton, Pixie Miller, Leah Koll, Tahvy, Kerry Spina, Elysha Emrich, Sequoia Glastonbury, Janelle Platt, Ali Schaffer, Jacqui, Charlotte Pointeaux, Mandy-Jane Hulse, Lora Love.

To all that I name here, and the countless people that shared the campaign within their networks, it was a humbling experience to watch the support blossom and you are all absolute legends in my book, pun intended!

Lastly I would like to honour Jay for holding the fort and looking after our children whilst I work. For encouraging me to go out to café's to write because you know it's bloody hard to focus with the incessant background noise of 4, sometimes 6 wildlings at home. You keep putting up with my cranky moods from so many late nights writing and the hours upon hours of research to print and distribute in the most efficient and ethical way. In my tiredness and wild creative flux, you have remained patient and for that I am grateful, because when you are my rock I can roll with the flow of it all and rest and replenish when needed.

PREFACE

Maiden is the first book in a series that speaks to the Sacred and spiritual nature of being a woman. The words that flow through my fingertips are offered with devotion and the intention of creating a beautiful legacy for my daughters, and theirs, and yours.

I have had the honour to sit with women in sacred circles and ceremonies that I've created and facilitated for over a decade, many of whom were or became mothers during this time. We often shared deep intimate conversations leading to discussions around the lack of resources for how to initiate young girls into womanhood. Sure there were books about puberty and 'moon time' wisdom, but nothing really offered a deeper perspective on how significant this time is.

After I free-birthed my 3rd daughter, I realised there was a reason my path lead me to learn and explore the women's mysteries. I was responsible for role-modeling and guiding 3 beautiful young girls into becoming embodied women. I wasn't actually planning on writing this book, in fact I started writing Maiden to Mother first, which shares my wisdom gained from the birthing field, but after I freebirthed my son Zenith in 2019, the 26,000 words I wrote on a weekend before he was born became an echo in the files of my laptop. As much as I wanted to delve back into the majickal creative process of writing that book, it was put on the back burner.

Then, in 2020 my eldest daughter began showing signs of approaching menarche. I had envisioned her ceremony and had been planning elements of that for years. It was an exciting time for me as a mother and after creating her beautiful menarche/maiden ceremony that I share in this book, I was asked by mothers around the world to share my wisdom and to create something that they could use as a practical guide.

It wasn't the first time I had been asked to do this. I thought I would create a new online course for the Wise Wombman Wisdom School and then I realised I needed to activate that rhythmic cadence of feverously tapped keys with wild, inspired writing. All of a sudden my creative vision was clear and in many sneaky moments of 10mins here and there, late nights with a cup of tea in hand and my son at the breast, I managed to write and complete my first book, Maiden. And here we are!

It's funny looking back now, and tuning into the stories I had playing out in my mind as to why I had not completed the other manuscript. Maiden. A Mothers Guide to Puberty and Menarche as a Sacred Rite of Passage was meant to be the first seed planted, the legacy birthed into the world, casting ripples of practical and spiritual wisdom, inspiration and guidance that will continue to blossom as do our young Maidens. I mean it makes sense; this book is about the sacredness of the womb and our blood. It is about the importance of understanding these sacred rites of passage that shape a young woman today, and the generations birthed through the portal of her womb. With awareness and loving presence we can lift the shackles of shame that have burdened young women around the world, across many different countries and cultures for far too long.

I trust that this guidebook will help to establish a worldwide legacy of initiating young girls into womanhood in such a way that speaks to each woman's soul with deep love, respect, compassion, creativity, beauty and reverence whilst also fiercely protecting the sweet essence and innocence of our young maidens.

Love Donna xx

INTRODUCTION

WHAT IS A MAIDEN?

In the patriarchal sense a Maiden is defined as a young female who is unmarried or a virgin.

In Pagan mythology, it pertains to The Triple Goddess, Maiden, Mother and Crone.

Maidenhood is synonymous with springtime and is symbolically tied to fertility and growth in many cultures. Think of the blossoming buds of spring, and how that relates to a young girl, slowly unfurling and emerging into the full bloom of womanhood.

The Maiden's initiation is through Menarche, Mother is through birth/creation and Crone is through Menopause. All are Sacred rites of passage that women embark upon during the different seasons of her life.

However, as society grew and changed, and the life expectancy became longer, many women did not feel completely represented in the triple goddess depictions. Where did women who were in their 40's, who had not undergone menopause fit in… and what about women who did not physically birth babies?

Based on the work of Elizabeth Davis and Carol Leonard's book, *The Women's Wheel of Life*, there are actually 13 seasons and archetypal expressions that speak to the natural rhythms and cycles of the female experience.

Our western consumer based society worships the season of the Maiden. From early teens to mid twenties, the season of the maiden is ripe with beauty, fertility, sexual receptivity and erotic innocence. Everywhere you look, from the billboards and magazines to the advertising of products, the young feminine form is celebrated and put on a pedestal of desirability.

This is deeply ingrained into our culture, and only a certain "type" of Maiden is given the platform and status as an icon, which perpetuates a false narrative of the Maiden, diminishing the vast array of gifts she has the capacity to give and narrowing her into the box of sexual desire, availability and fertility.

By only displaying a certain type of Maiden, it sets up subconscious programming to young girls that this is what is acceptable, this is what you should strive for, this is what we want, and if you don't fit it- then buy products to change your appearance, or do whatever you can to alter your appearance to become more desirable and compete in the "sexual marketplace".

It is very important to prepare your daughter to be able to identify and unpack this bombardment of subconscious programming, to nurture her ability to critically think, and to move through the teenage years with her self-esteem intact. Raising a generation of women who can see the game will empower them to decide if they want to play along or create a new world that fits their own creative capacity to be themselves fully embodied and giving other girls and women the inspiration to do so as well.

1

PREPARING FOR WOMANHOOD

*P*reparing young girls for menarche begins by demystifying the physiological process of bleeding. As a mother, you are able to share in the very normal and natural process of menstruation by allowing her to see your blood at an early age. This is as simple as her seeing you change a menstrual pad, and becoming familiar with your own cycle, showing and modelling to her that there is nothing to be ashamed about. Because there isn't!

DOING MOST of the groundwork before puberty enables the awkwardness to be limited because she has been guided to see the natural beauty of the menstrual cycle and how you relate to it. Exposing your daughter at an early age helps her to become comfortable with her own body as a woman. Think of it as an imprinting stage, a time of subtle education and preparation.

. . .

If you carry shame about your body and bleeding, your daughter will pick up on this subconsciously. A way to heal your own feelings of shame is to think of this as an initiation, not only for your daughter, but for yourself also. The wisdom contained in this book is offered as a guide and also part of your remembering. It is important that you embody the power and majick of your own menstrual cycle, so that you can pass your wisdom on.

The bonds of Mother to daughter are powerful, as they honour a direct link to the womb and creation energy. As you begin to heal any disconnect in yourself, you will help to create a powerful legacy as the Matriarch of your maternal line. What a gift for the future generations of daughters, and those connected to them. The first step is to become educated on your own cycle and to consider working with your blood in a ceremonial way. So keep reading, the information presented in this book is as much for you as it is your daughter.

Menarche is the first defining Blood Rite a young woman experiences. The second being sexual intercourse and third being birth, before the last as menopause. These rites are all centred around our Sacred Blood.

The first bleed is a powerfully symbolic and emotionally charged time in a young woman's life. During this sacred rite of passage she will be imprinted with sensory information, which will help her to establish and define who she is as a Sovereign being and cyclic woman.

The energetic signature of her first menses will follow her into these other blood rites. This young maiden energy will show up at the altar of birth and it is important to make this time as welcoming and natural as possible to free her from the taboo many cultures around the world have placed on bleeding women.

It is also important to note that other external influences around this time can be carried in the womb subconsciously, forming her foundations as a woman.

For example, I came to realise that I had a deep seated belief that being a woman meant to be in pain because my first bleed happened around an emotionally volatile time at home and it was physically excruciating. So much so, I was convinced I was going to die. Trauma effects individuals in different ways, and any trauma experienced as the womb is activating for the first time can anchor some powerful beliefs that may or may not be in the best interest of a woman connecting to self and her sensual nature. These beliefs can take years to reveal and heal.

Having said that, even if there was a missed opportunity for creating a beautiful experience, there is always a pathway for healing and connection, which can be done at any time one chooses. Simply recreate the rituals outlined further in the book.

ONE OF THE beautiful things about being a Mother of a daughter is that you are already innately qualified to help guide her into womanhood, because you yourself embarked on that journey. Even if you did not have adequate guidance, or you walked that journey blindly- the fact you have experienced the transition through menarche means that you know what it can be like, and you know that it can be different for your daughter. That is probably a big reason why you are reading this, because when you know better, you do better. Most women I know were not initiated in a way that was meaningful or Sacred, and I wonder what the world would look like now, if they had.

. . .

IMAGINE a world where each young woman was taught to honour and celebrate her body by having access to the language and wisdom of the womb from the beginning. Imagine how this would help shape her confidence around her cycle, and how empowered she would feel knowing her own physiological, mental, emotional and spiritual patterns as she develops a deeper connection to and with her womb.

IMAGINE a world where young women were taught to listen to their bodies, to rest and nourish themselves and know they are whole, as themselves. Imagine they felt comfortable and confident in all the different phases and expressions that come with being a cyclic woman.

IT IS important to mention that there is an insidious agenda at play by large corporations that prioritise profits over people. It is like a parasite that feeds off the impressionable psyche of a young girl in a bid to corrupt her capacity to critically think and question the status quo. It operates in very covert ways, constantly bombarding the subconscious with programs designed to corrupt innocence, creativity and sensuality by perpetuating unbalanced and often unrealistic models of femininity, which in turn create passive consumers bound with fear and deep sense of inadequacy.

I mention this because this season of Maidenhood, where our young girls are transitioning and blossoming into young women is such an important part of development and helping your daughter move through this, with her self-esteem and identity intact, in an age of fast paced technology and social media, is of utmost importance… its' almost an act of rebellion.

Professor and Radical Feminist, Gail Dines once said,

> *"If tomorrow, women woke up and decided they really liked their bodies, just think how many industries would go out of business"*

And this has always struck a resonant chord in my heart.

2

PUBERTY AS AN INITIATION

I had to look back at my own journey into womanhood, with the wisdom that I have now to replicate what was helpful, and fill in the gaps where I felt I was left in the dark- particularly because my home life and my parent's relationship was quite volatile at the time.

I distinctly remember when my breast buds began to develop, and feeling this small stone sized lump in my breast and thinking I was going to die of cancer. I was so shocked it actually sparred me into a bit of an existential crisis. I was certain I didn't have long to live, and I was unsure how to tell my family and share this burden of impending death. I was living at my dad's house and I remember my mum coming over to visit and when I told her, she laughed at me, saying it was just my mammary glands developing... and the little tomboy me was like, "huh?"

As my eldest daughter began to grow older, I started to prepare and educate myself on what other signs to look for which signified her body was in the transition phase. What I learned was that about a year or so before a young girl begins her menstrual cycle, you will begin to notice subtle changes of the onset of puberty. Of course this will vary for each individual.

Puberty is such an intense time of change, physically, mentally and emotionally. Giving your daughter some reference points of what to expect with these changes can help her transition into womanhood become something beautiful, symbolic and exciting.

When my eldest daughter was around the age of nine I began to speak to her about the changes her body would go through, and that her body had a unique intelligence and wisdom that would begin the process in its own timing. Over the following couple of years we would have conversations around puberty and the physical and hormonal changes that were inevitable.

Our relationship has been built upon communicating without shame, and bringing elements of humour into the spaces that create awkward tension. I had to remind myself what it was like to be so young, innocent and hungry for knowledge.

SOME OF THE signs to notice are the change in skin, with more blemishes or hormonal acne. Breast buds developing. Pubic hair. Body odour. Growing pains and disrupted sleep, or they are sleeping much more than usual. These changes usually go hand in hand with a big growth spurt or developmental leap.

Vaginal discharge usually begins 6-18 months before the onset of menses. I would always check my daughter's underwear when doing the washing for signs she was entering into this season, so I could make sure to start having more frequent conversations and prepare her menstrual gift basket, which you'll learn about in chapter 5.

I ALSO LET my daughter know to expect changes to her vulva in shape, labia size and pigmentation and to use a mirror and develop a connection with her genitals, educating her about the fact that there are so many variations to what vulvas look like, that the more she developed a relationship with herself in this way, then she would be able to map any changes that may be cause for concern.

I felt it was important to empower her with this knowledge, so that she did not feel any shame around her body, because I did when I was a teenager and it was such a horrible feeling to think that there was something wrong with you, when everything was actually healthy down there. I also felt it was important to teach her that her scent *'down there'* would change too, and that so long as her genitals did not smell foul or off or cause her physical pain, then everything was ok.

PUBERTY BRAIN

The brain goes through so many changes during the adolescent years. This is a time of rapid growth and is the time when the cerebral cortex (the outer layer of the brain that is used for reasoning and abstract thinking) begins to mature. As neuroscience has progressed over the years, we have been able to understand more fully what happens to the brain during puberty and understand the power of hormones. As a mother you would know how powerful these hormones are because you would have experienced the effects of them in various ways.

HORMONES

When my daughter was around the age of 9, I began to speak to her about hormones and the impact they have on our reproductive health and wellbeing. A very simple way for her to understand this was to witness the hormonal fluctuations in me as I was experiencing them. I shared with her that my skin would usually break out in a few pimples in lead up to my bleed, regardless of my diet.

She began to notice this physical change in me and ask me if I was due for my period. I would also share with her that during my ovulation phase I was more playful. Just before my bleed I would have a flux of energy and during my bleed I was more introverted and would seek warming foods and rest, sometimes sugary foods too.

Simple things like this helped to normalise the experience of being a cyclic woman. She began to formulate her own language around what being a woman was, and I wanted her to see it as a beautiful and empowering journey, because the stories we formulate in the early years can stay around for a long time and impact our way of thinking, feeling and being. Being open and transparent helped to prepare her for the more "heady" discussions around the role of our hormones, how they affect us, and warning signs when they are out of balance.

I felt it was important to let her know that she could anticipate changes in her body from puberty, as well as her mind because I believe that mental health and wellbeing should be treated in the same way as physiological wellbeing.

We talked about estrogen, progesterone and testosterone and how these affect the body. I shared how these hormones can sometimes make you feel lots of new and different emotions. I also talked about oxytocin, dopamine, serotonin, adrenaline and the impact of cortisol.

THE BEAUTIFUL PART about living in modern times is that we have access to a plethora of information right at the end of our fingertips. I don't suggest that you prepare a lecture on neuroscience, though I do feel it is helpful to plant these seeds and terms so that your daughter can follow up and research on her own. In doing so, she will learn more about how the chemicals in her brain can alter her experiences in life. This will also help to lift the stigma around mental health, so that she will be confident in seeking or asking for help if she feels she needs it.

MY MOTHER PREPARED me to expect a dramatic change in my thinking, hormones and mood and to look at puberty this way. I found it was beneficial to know this beforehand, to somehow buffer the confusion and intensity that came with puberty and the built up confusion and internal angst I started to feel. Mum knew I was in for a wild ride, being the baby of four children. I somehow missed seeing this in my older sister as there was a 7-year gap, so whilst she was going through puberty, I was still in the realm of majickal childhood.

. . .

Having a reference point for what to expect, without boxing me in, really helped me to explore and experiment with my newfound sexuality. It also helped me to know that my sleeping, mood, teen angst and attitude were all normal fluctuations of chemicals in my brain.

I still went through the, "nobody loves me, everybody hates me, maybe I'll go eat worms" victim cycle. I still back-chatted and dropped my head and shoulders back with a loud "UGH!" as teenagers do. There were still times where I hated the world and felt like everyone and everything was against me, times of contemplating suicide because the drama of highschool relationship dynamics were intense, but it was short lived.

Thank goodness!

I truly believe that when we empower our children with the knowledge of how things work and allow them to fill in the gaps, it helps to create strong emotional and mental resilience. We have to set them up for success and give them tools to navigate the times when life just sucks, because let's face it… sometimes it does!

MENARCHE: A RITE OF PASSAGE

Menarche is the first menstrual cycle, or first period of a female. Menarche is often considered a defining moment in a young girls life as she transitions into womanhood. It is a sacred rite of passage, which signifies the event of puberty and expresses the possibility of fertility. Girls experience menarche at different ages, the global average being around 12 years old.

Menstruation goes by many different names. Some of these are quite known and clinical like Menses and Period, whilst others are quite whimsical and comical, such as; Aunt Flo, P-plates, Red River, Rags, Lady Business, Moon Time, Crimson Tide, Shark Week, Leak Week, etc.

Etymologically related to the word Moon, menstruation and menses are derived from the Latin mensis, meaning month and Greek mene, meaning moon. So the roots in English point to moon and month.

IN SOME CULTURES a party or celebration is thrown to show the girl's transition to womanhood.

Today, we are now seeing a revival of honouring the first bleed as a Sacred Rite of Passage as a young girl officially and symbolically transitions into Maidenhood. More and more women are starting to connect with the womb as a Sacred space, healing any menstrual shame and becoming empowered by their blood. Women are starting to remember how to tap into the wisdom of the womb and using it to create with the energies of their cycle in a powerful and holistic way. It is because of this reclamation of the Sacred Womb, that mothers want to change the story, HERstory- the female and often-untold version of history, and rewrite a new beginning for the future generations of women who feel safe and powerful in their bodies and experience as a female.

THE REVIVAL OF CEREMONY AS A SPIRITUAL PRACTICE

Ceremony has been a powerful practice and the spiritual backbone of many different cultures throughout the human experience. It is the act of coming together in a symbolic way that honours, pays respect to, marks or signifies a specific event in a way that is meaningful to those engaged in the practice.

In some of the worlds most ancient cultures people celebrated the Earth's seasons and cycles as well as individual and collective's growth by way of Sacred Rites of Passage.

THE POWER of Ceremony lays in the impact it has on the human psyche as it creates the ability for us to step outside of the everyday mundane, and step into the realms of the mystical world with a shared experience of what is Sacred. Ceremony shifts us from one dimension to another, and during such, the man-made construct of linear time has no weight as you enter into the otherworldly realms of the timeless.

Whenever there is high emotion around something we tend to retain and store the sensory information in the form of memory. Through the activation of the limbic system, the part of the brain that is responsible for stored memory and emotion, ceremonies help to create powerful portals of meaning, as they are created with the intention to symbolically mark a significant time, event or rite of passage.

In the modern world, we have grown up with a complete disconnect to Sacred ceremony and individual rites of passage. Our standard reference points are birthdays, weddings, graduations and funerals but nothing that really speaks to or honours the evolution and maturity of an individual and the different seasons we go through in life, like coming of age.

However, we can draw upon the wisdom from those who have walked before us and begin to revive our connection to ceremony by becoming curious and creative in the ways that we acknowledge moments of significance. We can begin to look at ways to create meaning around transitions, endings, new beginnings and celebrating the beauty of our natural world and life itself.

CEREMONY HAS the ability to unite people into the present moment, with a central focal point of shared intention, mutual love and respect, whilst walking common ground together. It is a great way to connect with Spirit, Country, the custodians of the land and ancestral lineages. Paying respects and gratitude to all those who have walked before us, and those generations into the future that we will never get to meet.

OVERCOMING CULTURAL SHAME + STIGMA

Unfortunately, the majority of women today did not have a "sacred initiation" into womanhood. As a facilitator of women's circles and womb work for the last decade, I have been privy to hearing many women speak of their first blood in a way that was treated as an insignificant or traumatic event, a burden or something to be ashamed about. The monthly visit from *Aunt Flo* was often associated with pain, discomfort and dread.

. . .

IN MANY CULTURES around the world, a woman during her menses is considered dirty, unclean and is often removed, by self-isolation from the day-to-day duties, including work and schooling. In some places, a bleeding woman was not allowed to pray or enter places of worship and she could apparently spoil crops and produce.

Womb Blood was and still is taboo.

Something we don't talk about.

Something that is hidden out of sight, an inconvenience that just under half the population endures in silence.

THE WOMB, whilst revered for its service in creating new life, is cast aside for its cyclic nature. Just like the female body, if it is not productive in producing life or male pleasure, it is ignored. Although the roots run deep, this perspective is a product of our contemporary culture of consumerism that reduces women to body parts, and if they are not functioning correctly, they are not important to know about.

The myths centred around impurity can be traced through many cultures, and seem to have a narrative that has been twisted, misinterpreted or taken out of context which have then created a sub-culture of menstrual myths, perpetuating silence and shame, leading many women to be afraid of their blood, to see, touch or smell it.

This spin of perception may have derived from the fact

that in more ancient times, women would naturally take time off during their menses. It was actually revered as an important time of rest and renewal, and also when she was at the height of her intuitive capacity. Resting during this time allowed the women to tap into their primal and mystical wisdom that would help serve the family and community at large.

It seems more logical that women didn't enter the places of worship because they valued their rest and rejuvenation. Over time, this became misrepresented and thus created the story that woman could not enter the temple or practice her religious and spiritual ceremonies because she was considered "impure". Funnily enough, it is said that because of the domestic duties women uphold in their communities, like growing, birthing and rearing children, keeping house, cooking and tending to livestock, that women did not need to seek God, for God would naturally come to women.

THE VERY ESSENCE and nature of humanity derives from the blood of woman. So how can the blood that brings forth life be so impure and unholy? It makes no logical sense, though it has kept women "in their place" for generations- and not for the practice of rest and renewal. Other impurity myths simply stem from the fact that many women do not have access to menstrual hygiene products.

IN SOME COUNTRIES, (even in remote communities in Australia today) many young girls and women do not have access to feminine hygiene products, or are not adequately educated and empowered with the wisdom of the womb, resulting in many missing out on school, work, cultural events and developing severe health problems like sepsis.

We definitely have a "period privilege" in the capitalist modern world, in that we have easy access to menstrual products like pads, tampons, period pants, cups, sponges, etc. even though they are taxed as luxury items in some countries. It is important to take a moment to acknowledge that there are women today who are continually living with the shame of 'spoiling' their clothes and whatever resources they use to catch their blood, are things like cardboard, dirt, bark, ash or leaves.

I MADE it a point to educate my daughter on her privileges from an early age so that she could use them to help educate and empower other girls. Imagine a world where all young girls could bleed safely, freely and without shame or disruption to their education and employment opportunities.

3

REPRODUCTIVE / SEXUAL HEALTH AND WELLBEING

*I*t's not enough to simply share the beautiful side of menstruation, it is very important to begin to have conversations that centre on reproductive health and wellbeing. As most young girls who bleed are not (by their own choice) sexually active in their early adolescent years, these discussions can start out in an age appropriate "need to know" basis based on your connection and discernment. As a mother, it is imperative to set the SAFE space for your daughter to come to you for this wisdom because she may not receive it from school or her peers, or it may come through in a distorted way.

BE mindful that there may be an awkward tension in these moments. How you manage your state, will create the feeling of openness and reciprocity. It is important to see your daughter as a Sovereign being, on her own journey into womanhood trying to navigate this and the influx of hormones, so be gentle and allow the space for playful curiosity in questions- even if they make you feel uncomfortable and squirmy. She may be totally different to you and have a different perspective or communication style. Try to meet her where she is welcoming connection. If you don't have the answers to her questions, then simply welcome the opportunity to explore it together in researching, or finding an appropriate channel for the information she is seeking.

Encourage your daughter to connect with her developing body as a practice of self-care and general health and wellbeing. This is important, because the more she becomes in tune with her body, the easier it will be to notice any subtle changes that may be a cause for concern. I demonstrated to my daughter a simple breast/lymph massage that she could do in the shower and I spoke to her about using a mirror in the privacy of her bedroom to explore the features of her genitals in a way that would allow her to become familiar with her own body.

I talked to her about vaginal health and hygiene, the changes of the vulva during puberty, and that it's not just a bunch of pubes down there. We also spoke about her private parts being Sacred and we talked about pleasure, consent, boundaries and being able to say no- even if it hurts someone's feelings. I know she won't be sexually active for quite some time, yet these are important seeds to plant now so it becomes natural for her to respect her body.

Bringing humour into conversations helps to get to the teachable moments to anchor the information in a clear way. It's a much better approach than her resisting information because she feels awkward. Obviously, you need to pick your moments to educate and inspire, and let her lead the way by asking open ended questions that build's the conversation.

I AM so grateful that my mother held this space for me, to be curious and to know that I could ask her anything without judgement, or that I could come to her if I was unsure or needed advice. Knowing I had her there definitely had an impact on my sense of safety and being held- I also feel that it gave me the security I needed to experiment and explore my sexuality, yet not enter into too many risky situations because I had a reference point for what the consequences might be. To this day, my mother and I are very close because of the way she demonstrated her unwavering love and commitment to me becoming ME.

THE BIOLOGY OF THE MENSTRUAL CYCLE

On the outside, the basic biology of the female menstrual cycle appears to be simple, you bleed for a few days, then a week or so later you ovulate, and if no pregnancy occurs you bleed again. It all sounds so simple, yet it is actually a complex series of events that rely upon the healthy function of the hypothalamus, pituitary gland, ovaries and the endometrium (the thick lining of the uterus/womb).

THE FOUR PHYSIOLOGICAL phases of the menstrual cycle are menstruation, the follicular phase, ovulation and the luteal phase.

. . .

MENSTRUATION IS the shedding and elimination of the build up of thick lining of the womb (endometrium) through the vagina. Menstrual fluid contains blood, mucous and cells from this lining. The average length of a period is approximately 3 to 7 days and the first day of a menstrual cycle coincides with the flow of blood.

The follicular phase begins on the first day of bleeding and ends with ovulation, usually around day 10. During this time, the hypothalamus (controls the autonomic nervous system and regulates the pituitary gland's release of hormones that then stimulate other endocrine glands to release hormones) sends a signal to the pituitary gland to release FSH, Follicle Stimulating Hormone, which stimulates the ovary to produce follicles on the surface, sometimes up to 20 with each of these being home to an immature egg. No wonder we are born with so many eggs! In most cases, only one follicle will mature into an egg on the surface, while the rest die off. The growth of these follicles is what tells the womb to start producing the thick lining (endometrium), in preparation of supporting a pregnancy. It also causes a spike in estrogen levels, and once the hypothalamus recognises this, it will begin to release Gonadotrophin Releasing Hormone aka GnRH. This hormone triggers the pituitary gland to produce raised levels of LH, Luteinising Hormone and FSH.

Amazing huh? But wait… it gets more fascinating!

OVULATION IS the release of a mature egg from the ovary and is triggered by the high levels of LH. Once released from the ovary, the egg begins to make its way down the fallopian tube towards the womb. If unfertillised, eggs will die in approximately 24 hours.

The luteal phase happens during ovulation where the ruptured follicle stays on the surface of the ovary after the egg is released from it. The follicle then begins to transform into what is known as the Corpus Luteum, which starts releasing progesterone and small amounts of estrogen. This powerful combination of hormones helps the womb to maintain its thick lining while waiting for a fertilised egg to stick, which is known as implantation. If successful, the Corpus Luteum will continue to produce progesterone, which is needed to help maintain pregnancy as well as HCG, Human Chorionic Gonadotrophin. Higher levels of HCG is what is being tested for a positive pregnancy test via urine or blood.

If there is no pregnancy, the Corpus Luteum dies and the sudden drop in progesterone levels causes menstruation as the womb lining that has built up during this time begins to naturally shed and expel from the vagina, which starts and then repeats what we call the menstrual cycle.

HOW STRESS AFFECTS THE MENSTRUAL CYCLE

Cortisol is known as the stress hormone and is produced by the adrenal glands. Secretion of the hormone is controlled by the hypothalamus, the pituitary gland, and the adrenal gland, often referred to as the HPA axis. It usually signals the human brain to stop the release of reproductive hormones progesterone and estrogen. Both of these reproductive hormones are necessary in stimulating the menstrual cycle. Without these hormones, the menstrual cycle cannot occur.

Sudden or even prolonged stress can have a great impact on the reproductive hormones. It usually interferes with how the ovaries function in making progesterone and estrogen. Besides making your periods late, stress may also have effects on one's menstrual cycle in several other ways. This is important to know because stress can increase the chance of abnormal cycles, which can impact your health and wellbeing in various ways.

LATE AND ABNORMAL CYCLE

Growing up, we know that a late period can be an indicator of pregnancy, but what happens if you're not sexually active? I remember the first time I "flip cycled" going from bleeding on the full moon to bleeding with the dark moon and I wondered what was going on inside of me.

Late periods can happen when it takes a longer time for the eggs to ovulate. This can mean that the first part of the menstrual cycle will be much longer and the menstrual cycle shall be late (this is known medically as Oligomenorrhea). Bleeding can start about 12-14 days after ovulating as a result of the effects of stress levels on the reproductive hormones.

Missed periods can happen when the ovaries make less estrogen and so the womb lining doesn't not grow at all, which means there is nothing to shed. This is a more extreme result of stress known as hypothalamic amenorrhea. It's important to note that the stress can be emotional, environmental and physical.

Sometimes the eggs will grow and you will make enough estrogen, but you do not ovulate. The womb will shed it's lining but it might come very early or late, or have a stop/start quality leading to the experience of an irregular period. The bleeding depends on how much the womb lining has been stimulated by the estrogen produced.

CAUSE FOR CONCERN with abnormal cycles is if at any stage you intuitively feel something is not right. If your cycle is late due to low estrogen for more than 6 months it can actually begin the process of your bones thinning and the risk of osteoporosis increases.

WHEN RETROGRADE MENSTRUATION OCCURS, some blood and tissue flow backward up the fallopian tubes instead of forward and down through the vagina. If endometrial tissue clogs the fallopian tubes or reaches the abdominal cavity, inflammation and illness can occur. Common symptoms that can suggest this condition include stomach pain, soreness of the lower abdominal area, and cramping even after menstruation ceases. Experts suggest it is best to avoid inverted yoga positions that can affect the flow of blood.

1 IN 10 women who experience extreme period pain are actually experiencing symptoms of endometriosis which occurs when cells normally found in the lining of the womb begin to grow in other areas of the body, including the bowel, ovaries and even the lungs. These cells are shed every month in the same way that the womb sheds its lining, causing a period and it can take up to 7 or 8 years

for some women to be diagnosed and receive help. Wild! This is mainly due to a lack of awareness and education. Experts believe endometriosis is caused by genetics or a combination of genetics, estrogen dominance, oxidative stress and immune dysfunction. Women's quality of life can suffer dramatically from this debilitating and painful inflammatory disease.

This is the type of education our daughters need to feel empowered with their own health and wellbeing and also to be able to support their friends.

CYCLE MAPPING

The easiest and perhaps most important way to connect with the womb is to map the menstrual cycle as a way to understand yourself in an empowered way.

To encourage my daughter to begin her journey connecting with her womb space, I showed her the importance of mapping her menstrual cycle and then incentivised the process so that she actually WANTED to do it... by her own will and determination, not because mum told her so! We made a deal that she had to map her cycle for at least 1 year and 1 day, before she could fully receive her initiation gift that was bound to her menarche ceremonial candle, which you'll learn about in chapter 4.

By adding this element of challenge and reward, it helped her to stay focused to actually fulfill the process of mapping her cycle, the phases of the moon, her thoughts and emotions. She thinks the gift is a majickal ankh necklace, but the real gift will be the revealing of her own pattern and understanding herself more clearly. This gift is priceless!

. . .

I didn't start mapping my cycle until I was in my late 20's and by that stage I was already a mother of 2. Had I been given this wisdom as a necessary practice of empowerment, I may have been able to dodge hormonal birth control, and would have gained a clearer understanding on how to work with my cycle and optimise my offerings and work, rather than masking symptoms and pushing on through when my body was screaming at me to stop and listen!

There are many resources to use in mapping your cycle. It can be as simple as marking day 1 and your fertile days on a calendar with colour and personal symbols or going deeper into cycle wisdom by journaling or using technology like an app used on a smartphone or device.

If you are wanting to encourage your daughter to journal, or perhaps you would like to begin your initiation into your own cycle wisdom, I thoroughly recommend "Spinning Wheels" and the "13 Moons Journal: A Cycle Charting Handbook & Journal" by Jane Hardwicke Collings, founder of MoonSong and the School of Shamanic Womancraft. Jane is an incredible wise woman and mentor with experiential wisdom as a midwife and leader in the women's mysteries.

There is such great beauty, transpersonal growth and majick about sitting with pen and paper and being present to what is, however sometimes life can be in a state of flux and creating space to "drop in" can be challenging. This is where technology can be used to our advantage because you can tap into this Sacred Wisdom whenever it is convenient.

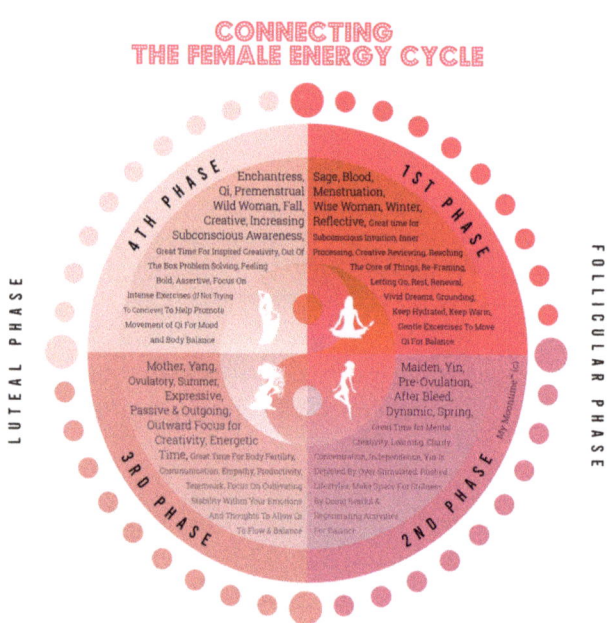

"MyMoonTime" is an affordable subscription based app made by females, for females.

Using technology is an efficient and powerful way to keep track of your menstrual cycle, be empowered with fertility awareness as well as living a life attuned to your natural rhythms so you can create a life of ease and flow.

According to the website, MyMoonTime "is one of the only period tracking apps that delivers physical and emotional forecasts so you can plan your life better, and be fully in sync with the forces that influence your ever-changing states."

EDUCATION LEADS TO EMPOWERMENT

Over the last decade, there has been an incredible movement happening worldwide which aims to lift the veils of shame around the menstrual cycle. Some of the most pivotal works that come to mind are as follows.

-Anita Diamant's book *The Red Tent*, written in 1997 shared a biblical fiction around women coming together in a menstrual hut and passing wisdom down to their daughters by initiation. Originally, the book did not do so well for shifting the perspective on menstruation, however by 2002, *The Red Tent* had become a New York Times bestseller and an international publishing phenomenon, selling over 2 million copies worldwide and pioneering a new wave of menstrual education which lead to the birth of the Red Tent Movement and many sacred women's circles around the world.

. . .

-Days for Girls Foundation, a non-profit organisation founded by Celeste Mergens in 2008. On their website, it states that the Days For Girls Foundation, "Increases access to menstrual care and education by developing global partnerships, cultivating social enterprises, mobilizing volunteers, and innovating sustainable solutions that shatter stigmas and limitations for women and girls."

Today, they have helped over 1.7million women and girls in 125+ countries with their menstrual hygiene kits and education. Revolutionary!

- In 2009, Eve Ensler's *The Vagina Monologues* took the stage by storm, exposing the stories of women she had interviewed around many topics at the forefront of the female experience, including the piece called "I Was Twelve, My Mother Slapped Me: a chorus describing many young women's and girls first menstrual period". Eve's work was paramount in giving voice to the silent pain, shame and struggle of women, to the point that in 2018 the New York Times stated, "No recent hour of theatre has had a greater impact worldwide".

-In 2015, artist Rupi Kaur was censored by Instagram for posting their menstrual art series *Period*. Kaur critiqued the social media platform's position by writing: "Thank you Instagram for providing me with the exact response my work was created to critique… I will not apologize for not feeding the ego and pride of misogynist society that will have my body in an underwear but not be okay with a small leak, when your pages are filled with countless photos/accounts where women . . . are objectified, pornified, and treated less than human." Consequently, Instagram reversed their decision, and menstrual art has since found a way to be expressed freely without censorship. #menstruation # period #periodart

- THE 2019 ACADEMY AWARD Winning Best Documentary Short, Period. End of Sentence. Focused on a rural village in India and helped to break the silence and taboo about female reproductive health and hygiene.

- 2019 MENSTRUAL PRODUCT COMPANY, Libra, aired their *#BloodNormal* ad in Australia that aims to normalise periods by showing red liquid on a pad, a woman in red stained underwear, a woman with blood trailing down her leg in the shower and a man picking up a packet of sanitary pads from the shop. This was revolutionary in the advertising arena, which previously used a blue liquid to demonstrate absorption of the sanitary products.

- IN HER 2020 TED Talk titled *"Why can't we talk about periods?"* gynaecologist and author Jen Gunter explains the damage of menstrual shame, subsequently leading to harmful misinformation and mismanagement of pain. In her educational talk, she declared the era of the menstrual taboos over and stated that, "It shouldn't be an act of feminism to know how your body works".

BOOKS TO EDUCATE AND INSPIRE

When my daughter was around 10 years old, I gave her a copy of the book called

Reaching for the Moon, by Lucy H. Pearce. This beautiful little book spoke to my daughter in a way that made all the subtle training and imprinting make sense. It was very special to see her light up and begin to understand the majickal journey she was embarking on, as she began to anticipate her first bleed with excitement and curiosity.

I THINK it's important to have a few different resources available for your daughter to peruse through in her own time as a way of initiating her quest for wisdom that helps her fulfil the prophecy of her being.

SOMETIMES WE CAN BE TOLD the same thing several times by the same person, and then someone comes along and says it in a slightly different way and it finally lands. This is what *Reaching for the Moon* did for my daughter and I am so grateful it found its way into my bookshelf- as if it were by Divine intervention. It is important as a mother, to read different wisdom around the menstrual cycle as a way of cultivating your own embodied wisdom and spiritual practice, which you can then share with your daughter.

MENSTRUATION BOOKS:

- ***Thirteen Moons & Spinning Wheels*** by Jane Hardwicke Collings
- ***A Blessing Not a Curse*** by Jane Bennett
- ***The Optimized Woman & Red Moon*** by Miranda Gray
- ***The Wild Genie*** by Alexandra Pope
- ***Women, Hormones and the Menstrual Cycle: Herbal and medical solutions from Adolescence to Menopause*** by Ruth Trickey
- ***Moonrites*** by Spiraldancer
- ***The Women's Wheel of Life*** by Elizabeth Davis and Carol Leonard
- ***Women's Bodies, Women's Wisdom*** by Dr. Christiane Nothrup
- ***Blood, Bread & Roses: how menstruation created the world*** by Judy Grahn
- ***The Wise Wound: Myths, Realities & Meanings of Menstruation*** by Penelope Shuttle & Peter Shuttle.
- ***The Period Book: A Girl's Guide to Growing Up*** by Karen Gravelle
- ***Period Power*** by Maisie Hill
- ***Period Queen*** by Lucy Peach
- ***Period. End of Sentence: A New Chapter in the fight for Menstrual Justice*** by Anita Diamant and Melissa Berton

EDUCATIONAL WEBSITES

- https://sexedrescue.com
- https://moonsong.com.au
- https://www.menstruationresearch.org/
- https://www.periodlove.com/
- https://www.menstrupedia.com
- https://www.bepreparedperiod.com/
- https://theperiodstore.com/
- https://blog.gladrags.com/
- http://www.theperiodblog.com/
- https://www.yoni.care/en/
- https://redschool.net/

MENSTRUAL APPS FOR ELECTRONIC DEVICES

- MyMoonTime
- Flo health
- P Tracker
- Clue
- Cycles

4

MAIDEN/MENARCHE CELEBRATION CEREMONY

ASKING PERMISSION

*C*onsent is key, especially at this season of growth. Whilst you may have this incredible idea about a Maiden Ceremony, it is really important to check in with your daughter to see if she is open to what you have in mind. You don't have to share all the details with her, but sharing the essence of how you want to celebrate her will help her to trust that it wont be embarrassing or weird.

I have 3 daughters, and I know that the ceremony I created for my eldest which I've documented in this book, may not be something my second born would resonate with. This event is about honouring and celebrating your daughter in a way that she can and will actually be open to receive. There is no point putting all the effort and resources into creating something that she will retract from.

. . .

KNOWING what *love language* your daughter connects with will provide valuable insight into what she values and how she appreciates being loved. This will give you a great focal point to really amplify the area of love being poured into the moment- whether that is words of affirmation, quality time or gifts in the blessings ceremony etc. You can find out more about love languages by browsing the internet or purchasing the book, "*Love Languages*" by Gary Chapman.

YOU MAY HAVE SEEN some fun ideas on *pinterest* for a period party, vulva cakes and red everything. It's important to know that she welcomes the ideas and any documentation, because you want to do whatever you can to elicit a sense of comfort and connection whilst minimising any sense of shame or embarrassment. Think about what wholesome energy you want these memories to imprint and then go from there. You do not have to "keep up with the Joneses" or follow the crowd. This is about allowing the opportunity for your daughter to feel connected, safe and honoured as a young woman and that may actually mean that you do something private and special together that is simple and low key.

FORTUNATELY, my eldest was all for ALL the things, and so I can share with you what we did, and also some other ideas that would work too. This is to help you create your own ceremony template and potent memories that you will both treasure for years to come. Above all else, trust the little whispers from your heart of what to create.

THE POWER OF RITUAL

A Ritual is a sequence of events performed in a symbolic way, with specific words, objects and activities. They follow a set structure and narrative and can help to connect with sacred rites of passage in all seasons of life- from birth to death and everything in between. Rituals are performed by those participating in it and are not bound or limited to when they can be performed. Although similar, a Ceremony is usually reserved for a special occasion, date/season etc.

CEREMONIES CAN BE ritualistic in nature, however they can have a number of people present, such as guests or witnesses who do not actually participate in any formal role of the performance of the ceremony.

TO PREPARE for any significant personal ritual it is important that you cleanse your body, mind and your ceremonial space. If you have a bath, then consider soaking in salts and majickal herbs, and working with your breath to really soften into your body with full presence. This includes your daughter in the lead up to her special day.

NEXT PREPARE YOUR SACRED SPACE, set up your altar and majickal tools. Think of the outcome so you can prepare for anything that you may need. This is important because it will allow you to completely immerse in the experience and process, rather than getting to an important step and realising you forgot something, like tissues or a lighter, which can disrupt the flow

Write out your intentions. Make it clear. Create your own scripts if you need to. Whatever will help you facilitate with confidence. You can use the Notes section in this book to outline a plan and then fine tune it later.

SETTING THE SPACE

Creating Sacred space begins with having a clear intention for how you are going to use the ceremonial space in a way that helps transport people out of the mundane and into a 'time out of time' so to speak.

You really don't need much; I know not everyone will have a *womb temple* at home, so work with what you've got and don't stress too much. The essentials for any ceremonial space, particularly of this nature, is to make sure it is private, physically and energetically comfortable, accessible to guests and suitable to the time of year you are gathering. Always have a back up option in place if you are going to be outdoors because you don't want to be limited in what you do because of the weather.

Think about entry/exit into the physical space and also where the sun rises and sets as it may be important to your spiritual and cultural practices. In some cases you may need to be granted permission by elders to access a certain area of cultural significance and to practice ceremony.

THE DÉCOR you choose is to help provide comfort and to enhance the aesthetics of your space. Introducing the colour red into the space by making use of red tapestries, cushions, candles, flowers, and art will help to symbolise the Sacred blood and the womb itself. You may prefer to use neutral tones, or white/black with accents of red, again this is totally up to you and what you feel your daughter will enjoy.

Use lighting, crystals, trinkets, talismans and foliage to beautify the space. Make it feel welcoming and intimate. Let the space speak to and compliment your daughter's personality; you may have to remind yourself that this is not about you so to speak, you have to keep your daughter at the forefront of your mind with the intention of creating a beautiful ceremony that acknowledges her initiation into womanhood.

Use oils and different aromas to create a sweet and welcoming ambiance. This is a powerful way to activate the limbic brain, which is necessary for potent ceremonial experiences.

WHAT IS AN ALTAR?

Traditionally speaking, an altar was a table or platform where there were different offerings in consecration or communion with the Divine, God or higher power. It was a place designed for worship, honour, connection and a point to create offerings to these spiritual energies and deities of cultural importance.

As a sacred space in and of itself, an altar has the function of altering the environment, both the physical energetic space and the psychological.

We are actually surrounded by so many different altars everyday, if we choose to see them as such. Like your bed for instance, could be perceived as an altar of intimacy where you offer your dreaming, lovemaking and most vulnerable moments of surrender.

Your kitchen bench/stove top becomes an altar where you prepare offerings for your sacred vehicle, where you honour Mother Earth for her bountiful gifts.

The family dinner table becomes an altar of connection and gratitude.

Guided by the power of intent, the altar helps to activate and amplify the spiritual energy of the space and ritual ceremony.

HOW TO CREATE YOUR MENARCHE ALTAR

If you are planning on sitting in circle, it is always beautiful to have your altar in the centre of the circle as it will be the central focal point and place of connection for those present.

There is no right or wrong way to create your altar as far as placing physical items goes. It all comes down to your intention. So connect with that first, and then follow your intuition to what feels beautiful to create; you might like to do this together as a way to connect and bond before the ceremony begins.

Use any sacred objects that are meaningful and provide beauty into the space. Perhaps a photo of her, or you both together would be a nice touch. Think of things that are symbolic with Maidenhood, fertility and the womb. Think flowers, crystals, candles, offerings, artwork, poetry, fruits, jewellery, oils, etc. You may wish to mark out the four cardinal points, North, East, South and West or add in anything else that is culturally significant and speaks to your lineage and ancestors.

For Auraura's Menarche Ceremony, I felt called to keep it really simple. I had a tray with 3 pillar candles at different heights, symbolic for Auraura, Myself and my Mother…Maiden, Mother and Crone. This was surrounded with scattered clear quartz crystals and silk rose petals. Simple and beautiful!

To the side of the circle space was a larger candle that was symbolic of the ancestral womb lineage, honouring all those women that have walked before us. With prayers it was lit when we started to activate the space, and when we began ceremony, my mother lit her candle from the ancestral candle. I lit mine from hers, and Auraura lit her candle from mine. This created a respectful flow from womb to womb to womb and honours the fact that the egg that created Auraura was present in my womb as I was growing inside of my mother's.

5

MENARCHE RITUAL IDEAS

BLESSING + GIFT

*H*aving a blessing ritual in the Menarche Ceremony is such a beautiful way of deepening the bonds of whoever is present by weaving them into the inner circle of the Maiden's world. It is a powerful way to demonstrate that she is not alone, and has the opportunity to reach out to other women when she feels she needs to call upon their wisdom and guidance.

Each woman reads or shares a blessing from their heart or a prayer for the Maiden's initiation into womanhood. The blessings can also offer memories of being witness to her growing from a young child and can offer experiential wisdom that is relevant and uplifting. It is important that the blessings shared are spoken with deep love and encourage the space of honesty and real connection from woman to woman.

After the blessings are read in the circle setting, a meaningful gift is presented. The nature of the gift is up to the giver, though it does not have to be of material wealth. It can be deeply symbolic of the gift of an experience together.

Some examples of appropriate Menarche gifts are as follows;

Oracle /Tarot cards, jewellery, candles, essential oils, crystals, ochre, anything from the natural world that is taken with permission and evokes a sense of beauty, a day out at a café, clothing, underwear, journal, books, anything that is relevant to your daughters interests.

RITUAL MENSTRUAL CANDLE

Candles are a beautiful tool to use in spiritual practice to set the mood and ambiance of the ceremony space. They help to charge and cleanse your Sacred space and can deepen the connection to your intention in a way that you can direct your energy to whatever you are focusing on with a deep presence.

I absolutely LOVE candles and what they gift to the space. I also love to make my own out of rolled beeswax, and sing my intentions and prayers into them as I create different sizes and shapes.

The idea of a menstrual candle is to gift your daughter with a practical tool that can help her connect with her monthly bleed in a ceremonious way, bringing presence to each cycle and the wisdom it brings.

Adding a candle ritual into the Menarche Ceremony is a beautiful way to flow between different segments. As part of my daughters initiation into the blood mysteries, I gifted her "*13 Moons and Spinning Wheels*" journal by Jane Hardwicke Collings which helps to create strong foundations of charting and mapping the menstrual cycle and emotions.

To set the intention for my daughter to become empowered by her body and its natural rhythm, we created a rolled candle that she could light for a few moments every month for 13 moons as a way to symbolically connect with the majick of her menstrual cycle and to create the space for her to tune in and listen beyond the noise of daily life. Setting strong foundations for her own spiritual practices as she matures.

In majickal traditions, a student wishing to study new practices will immerse themselves in the teachings for 1 year and 1 day as part of their initiation. Now, this may not actually happen in her first years of bleeding, and that is ok. Intention is everything and we can only encourage and trust the seeds that have been planted. I mention this because I don't want any mothers feeling upset if the consistency wanes as if it's somehow a failed task. It's not. Your daughter will reach for theses methods of spiritual practice if and when she is ready, and approaching it this way makes it a more empowering journey for her as she figures it out in her own way, in her own time.

HOW TO CREATE YOUR ROLLED CANDLE

If you are going to make your own rolled beeswax like I share in the ceremony images, I have found that using hemp or waxed cotton for the wick works well.

Using natural beeswax is best, so please steer clear of paraffin wax (made from petrochemicals and is usually what you find in discount stores) because it is toxic – you can tell this because they burn off black smoke and can often leave a residue on surfaces.

You can purchase rolled beeswax sheets online or try

and source locally. They are around 40x20cm and will make 1 decent sized candle that stands on its own. You will need a natural fibre twine for the wick, cotton or hemp work really well. Cut a strand of your twine to fit the smaller side, allowing for 1-2cm to protrude from the top, where you will light the candle. Place the strand to the edge and slowly roll the wax over the string to create the centre. You want to apply firm pressure to start with to keep the wick in place, but after it has been rolled once and secured, you only need to apply gentle pressure to roll the candle.

In ceremony you pass the wax around the circle so each woman has a turn to connect with the wax and their intention and roll the candle a little before passing it on to the person beside them. If it is an option, I would suggest that you start with the grandmother and then finish with Mother, before passing it back to the Maiden for completion. This is to honour linage and legacy.

You can also dress the candle with essential oils and majickal herbs, which is perfect if you do not have access to beeswax sheets. Use the same principle as above, whereby each woman connects with the candle, taking turns to dress it, anointing it with her prayers and blessings.

As part of Auraura's initiation gift, we also passed a special amulet around the circle- which was hidden in everyone hands. Each woman then bestowed her blessings and breath onto the pendant with their eyes closed. When it made its way to Auraura, she also, without knowing what it was, held it to her heart and blessed the pendant before wrapping it around the candle. She then opened her eyes to reveal the ceremonial candle as was then told the directions of usage; that it was to be lit at the start of her cycle each month as a way for her to stop, take a moment to check in with herself and what she is feeling to take stock of her emotions and to explore her needs. Once she had done this for 13 consecutive moons, or 1 year and 1 day, she would then be gifted her pendant that was wrapped around it with the red thread from circle.

TIME CAPSULE

A super fun way to create majick is with a time capsule. This can be a stand alone ritual, or your could place the written blessings inside as a way of completing the ceremony. What is beautiful about having handwritten blessings is that a lot of change can happen in the years that the time capsule is left to be, whether it is buried or kept in a closet. Some elders may pass on, relationship dynamics change, people grow... what a beautiful snapshot in time to have their handwriting on paper.

Another beautiful idea is to have your daughter write to her future self, sharing what she's feeling now, what's happening in her world, how she is feeling as a young Maiden. A digital letter can also be sent via futureme.org where it will store and then send you your email at the selected date. Without being too morbid, if you are going to have a time capsule for your daughter, I feel it is important that you let a couple of trusted people know where it is and at what time in the future it is to be opened. In the event that you are unable to be there, your daughter will still be able to receive her blessings.

I've created a few time capsules over the years and what I have found works really well for burial is plumbers pipe with 2 screw on end caps. It will create a lock tight safe for the contents inside. If you are burying the time capsule, you'll need to think ahead. Is the property you are on going to be accessible in years to come? It's important to think about placement so that if you were to move on, there would be minimal disruption to retrieve the time capsule after gaining permission to dig up the soil from the new caretakers or owners. This also goes for places out in nature. You will also need to make sure the spot is marked in some way. You can use GPS coordinates or simply pace from a solid landmark like a rock or tree… or even place something heavy over the spot that becomes part of the landscape.

SPIRAL LABYRINTH

If you have the space to do so, you can create a spiral or labyrinth using anything on hand to define the path. This could be rock, anything botanical, cloth, candles, garden hose, or simply carve it into the ground or sand. In the centre of the Spiral or Labyrinth stands Mother or Grandmother waiting with a blessing and a special gift in her hands. The young Maiden takes her time and walks with a gentle rhythm into the centre to receive acknowledgement and a coming-of-age gift. Upon walking out of the spiral or labyrinth, she does so with a newfound sense of being in the world as a young woman. You could have Mother or friends at the exit to acknowledge and celebrate her with flowers, welcoming her into the world of woman.

SHARED ARTWORK

A beautiful way to facilitate an intimate moment together is to share in the creation of an artwork or craft. This can be done as a group or one-on-one. Use the time to share stories, ask questions and talk about things that are a little taboo or strange. Open up discussion of body image, pleasure, sensuality, how awkward puberty can be. Share your stories in a way that is humourous, so that it lifts any tension that might be present.

The more open and relaxed you are, the more your daughter will soften and relax too. You might like to create a couple of pieces of artwork, the focus is not on the end result of a finished piece, the focus is on being present with your daughter whilst you create something together.

You might like to include a small artwork into the time capsule too. You could even use this time to create and sew cloth menstrual pads from fabric she has chosen beforehand, or maybe a special bag that could be used instead of a menstrual basket and then becomes a family heirloom, passed on to each daughter who can then add onto it when her time comes. Can you imagine what that would feel like to feel connected to a lineage of women who have created these rituals, even more powerful if you are the Matriarch that starts these new traditions for your family.

GUIDE STONES

The idea of the guide stones is so that the Maiden receives words of wisdom from the inner circle of women in her life. Each stone is written with a word or phrase to help guide the young maiden and to remember simple self care practices as she continues her journey blossoming into womanhood. She can then use them as she would oracle cards, choosing a stone each day; or she could use them to decorate her own altar, garden or place that honours her menstrual rituals.

How to create the guide stones in ceremony?

I purchased a small bag of flat glazed stones from the local hardware store along with a packet of coloured permanent markers. The stones were around 6cm in diameter and were not that heavy. Using the permanent markers, each woman collected a few stones and wrote helpful messages and words of wisdom on them. Guidance that centred around self-acceptance, creativity, self-love and nourishment are always healthy reminders for young women. Such as:

DANCE
> Love yourself
> I am enough
> I am beautiful
> Drink water
> Move your body

AN ALTERNATIVE to this is to create your own affirmation oracle cards. Simply choose how many you want to create, what size and shape and get creative on paper. Use any mediums for your desired look and simply laminate the paper when you're ready, trimming the edges of the cards to make sure there are no sharp bits left. Ideally you would want them to be easy to hold and stack together. This could be included in the shared artwork project where your guests contribute to the creation of the deck.

FLOWER CROWNS

What better way to celebrate the season of Maidenhood then creating a beautiful flower crown and adorning your blossoming daughter! Flowers can be sourced from your garden, purchased locally or you could ask any guests to bring a small bunch along to contribute to the crown. There are many ways to make a crown but what felt easiest to work with was florists/gardener's wire. The wire helped to create the structure of the crown so that the flowers could be woven into it, without then becoming too heavy. It also saved a lot of time. Recently I noticed my local craft store Spotlight, stocking some moss lattice amongst the popular terrarium supplies, this would also make a great base for the crown. You can also purchase material or silk flower crowns online which are quite beautiful too!

WEAVING THE WOMB WEB- THE RED THREAD

The Red Thread is a powerful symbolic tool that can be used in many different circles and in different contexts. It represents the sacredness of blood and the connection to the womb, something that unites women across all generations and timelines. The string is symbolic of the womb grid and the invisible web that weaves all women together in solidarity of sisterhood.

Whilst sitting in circle, the Maiden passes the string to the woman sitting next to her, who will then share a blessing. In Mother blessing ceremonies, a bead would be used, but in the setting of a Maiden circle, once the string is "charged" with blessings it is then wrapped around the ritual candle so that all the blessings and wisdom of the women present are activated each month when she lights her candle.

Alternatively, she can use the string for a craft project or something that has deep meaning and significance. The string could also be used to tie (loosely) around a menarche tree or plant, if that is something you choose to do. You could also use cotton that can then be used to sew part of her menstrual hygiene products.

RED STAINS AND OFFERINGS

Looking towards the natural world for inspiration, you can draw upon plants and minerals with natural dye qualities to incorporate them into simple rituals that honour the red thread, womb and connection to these sacred blood rites. Beetroot can be cut in half to stain the hands or skin upon being welcomed into circle. You can also create a stamp out of it to stain material used for craft projects like affirmation flags.

Henna can be used to adorn the body or womb in a decorative and symbolic way. Pitaya or dragonfruit can be used in a nourishing face-mask as it is full of antioxidants. Ochre can be used to paint the skin and anoint with words of deep meaning as it offers the grounding qualities of the Earth. Pomegranate, a tart red fruit bursting with juicy red jewels can be used as an altar offering as it carries codes connected to the Goddess. Red wine can also be used as an offering to give thanks to the Goddess and the abundance the Earth brings us.

The rose is perhaps one of the most well known

symbols representing the Divine Feminine. Aside from it being a high vibrational plant used in sacred ceremonies around the world, red roses can be incorporated into the ceremony space, especially rose buds that are just starting to open. Rose petals are always a nice touch to bring beauty and fragrance to the space and can be scattered around the altar, used to create an aisle or pathway or simply shower your young maiden with rose petals to welcome her into womanhood.

TAKING ADVANTAGE OF TECHNOLOGY

If you have important people that you would like to include in your ceremony, you can use technology in creative ways to create connection and meaning. From prerecorded messages and videos to live streaming video calls, there are ways to include people even though they can't be physically present.

You can also think of creative and theatrical ways to have them participate in some of the rituals, bringing added humour and sweetness to the circle. For instance, Auraura's grandmothers walked her into the ceremonial space, but if your daughter's family is not present, perhaps a video call could serve the same purpose and your daughter walks with a device into the space. You may need extra planning to make sure the participant has the resources they need beforehand, to create whatever is needed so that they have enough time to prepare and send by post.

PHOTO SHOOT.

I am fortunate that my best friend is the incredibly talented visionary photographer, Chanel Baran and that I was able to hire her to document Auraura's ceremony to share with you and the world. Whilst you may not be inclined to have your private ceremony documented in such a way, I do feel that it is a beautiful opportunity to book a photo shoot with a professional photographer or a close friend who can take images for you. Most smartphones these days have great lenses and take great quality photographs. Investing in some beautiful images of this special time, whether it's just your daughter or you have them taken together will provide precious memories for years to come.

HEALING YOUR OWN MAIDEN

As you begin to watch your daughter blossom you may begin to experience subtle or uncomfortable sensations in your body as unpleasant memories can begin to surface. If you have experienced a traumatic initiation into Maidenhood or are a survivor of sexual abuse, especially around the same age, then witnessing the innocence of your daughter and her transition can trigger a complex post-traumatic stress response. I say response because I am a firm believer that it is not a disorder and it is a very natural way of responding to deep trauma, where the charge is still felt in the body.

It is a fine line to walk between protection and projection, and part of keeping your daughter safe it to alleviate her from the weight of your own pain. If this happens, first and foremost it is very important to seek the support you need to manage these triggers in a safe, holistic and empowering way so that you protect your daughter from your past and eliminate the potential to project the pain of your story on to hers. It is such a courageous act to walk this particular path as a mother in this way, and I have the utmost respect for you as a fierce mother who can hold this space as a cycle breaker so they or the next generation can be free.

Healing your Maiden is inner child work, dialled in to the season you began to experience physiological changes. It is an opportunity to hold ceremony for yourself, to create the safety and connection that you may have needed during that time… to share the wisdom that you know now, and hold that younger version of yourself close, wrapping her up in your arms, laughing with her, sharing wisdom with her and most importantly loving on her and telling her how worthy she is of love, respect, kindness and all the beauty in the world.

You can create a Menarche ceremony for yourself and your girlfriends, make an event out of it, or you can sit in a quiet place for your inner journey work through journaling and visualisation practices, whatever is your way of connecting with that younger version of yourself and giving her what she needed, because she didn't know at the time, but you do now, because you lived it and survived. In this way, you can mother yourself into healing and freedom.

If there were traumatic events around your menarche, you can use emotional alchemy practices, like my Womb-Song practice to release any stuck or discordant energy that is dormant in the womb, and then begin to dream in a new reality, re-writing the old one. If you've traversed into the Autumn season of womanhood of Maga, through menopause, this is a great opportunity to call in healing of your blood rites. You can simulate blood with natural reds such as beets, berries or ochre and use them in sensual play to connect with your inner maiden through art and ritual that is intuitive in nature, because during this time, woman is very powerful in accessing her inner wisdom, before she steps into her Crone season to offer her gifts outwards into the community.

MENSTRUAL BASKET

For the past few years before my eldest began bleeding, I had been slowly building up special, significant and symbolic things that would be gifted to her in a menstrual basket. If you are not in the most stable financial position, this will help as you can purchase things gradually. If you're crafty, you could also make or wave the basket yourself to make it extra special and meaningful.

I wanted the basket to represent a welcoming gift, something that was to be treasured, yet also practical.

The day after her bleed, I had some one-on-one time with her in the afternoon and took her down to the river to connect and enjoy the afternoon sun. This was special because as the eldest of four, our time together is precious and rare.

I placed a towel over her basket so she could not see what her gift was, though she knew I had something special planned. As we arrived at the riverbed, I asked her to sit quietly cross-legged and feel into her body, to focus on all the different sensations present in the moment as she softened into her body and breath.

I began to set up around her, so that when she opened her eyes, she would see the gift before her.

Inside the basket:

- **Mense Sense** teen starter cloth pads + wet purse
- **Modi Bodi** period-proof pants (RED label for teenagers)
- Menstrual cup (instead of tampons)
- Organic cotton disposable pads and liners
- Favourite chocolates
- Fresh flowers
- **Clary Calm** essential oil blend (this is a dōTERRA blend)
- Red tealight candle
- Small Moroccan bowl for blood offerings

The gift basket was focused on more of the practical tools she would need, as I wanted to keep the more mystical side of things for her Menarche Ceremony, as she was welcomed into the Women's Mysteries with the red thread. The basket was symbolic of the womb and I wanted it to help her connect with blood being a gift of the womb.

Needless to say, Auraura was blown away by the care and the fact that I had "all bases covered". She felt more than prepared to move forward on her journey as a blossoming young woman.

As we were leaving, I really wanted to capture the moment, as this first bleed has such a wild innocence to it- hard to describe, but it was such a sacred time for me to witness as her mother, as if I was transported back in time acknowledging my own transition and that of the women who walked before me.

In this moment, witnessing the wild innocence of my 12 year old daughter, I could sense her excitement and anxiety and a taste of anticlimax as she realised she was finally "there".

HONOURING NEURODIVERSITY

How do you facilitate ceremony when your daughter, or family member is Neurodivergent?

I've had the pleasure of interviewing several mothers of daughters on the Spectrum to gain a deeper understanding of what this could look like, because it is often not spoken about in contemporary menstrual resources, which have a more neurotypical focus.

Of course, every child is different and it is common sense to first gain consent to create a special ceremony and to also ask what she would like. There is no point creating something that YOU want, because it may lead to disappointment, unnecessary stress and anxiety. Always think about what SHE would want, love and appreciate, because this is a very significant event in her life and will set the theme of what it means to be a woman.

When conversing with the different mothers, one common theme that presented itself was that it was important to have enough lead in time to make sure your daughter is comfortable with what you are planning, to limit the element of surprise and to create a sense of familiarity in advance. This also includes any books, gifts or menstrual products that can be used and tested from a sensory standpoint. Your daughter may need some time with her menstrual products to get used to the texture and sensations, including the sounds and smells associated. In this way, by the time her blood actually begins to flow, it wont be so overwhelming and you can focus on any other sensations that are present in her body that are new and that she may need guidance in coping with and understanding.

You know your daughter and how she responds to new information and sensory input, ask her what she would like. Perhaps she may feel more comfortable with being gifted the practical tools months in advance, rather that the day of her bleed. If she is non-verbal, you can look for her cues to show her interest or lack thereof. This can be handy when choosing pads, whether they are disposable or cloth ones. Perhaps you may have a fabric selection she can choose from in her own way, and then you can have them made into pads for her, making them more personal, special and familiar.

Normalising the natural process and function of menstruation at an early age is paramount to edifying all young girls into the power of menstruation without shame. It is beneficial to have low-key conversations about periods like it's no big deal and to include your daughter. One mother offered an example of how she connected with her daughter by saying, "'Hey, what should we do to prep for your period when you get it? It could be a while, but we might as well get you some things you might need."

I really love this gentle initiation as it helps the daughter maintain her autonomy and includes her in the decision making process.

One mother mentioned that a blessing gift be relevant to her 'special interests', and not so much symbolic to the menstrual cycle. I found this a beautiful way to really create a deep and meaningful moment of honouring your blossoming daughter.

All in all, you really need to work with what is going to help connect with your daughter in an empowering way and reduce any possible sensory overload or anxiety.

You may need to fully scale back the maiden ceremony, if that's what she wants.

You may need to come up with an idea together that she feels comfortable in receiving.

At the end of the day, ceremony is about intention and presence. You do not need all the bells and whistles to make it deeply meaningful and symbolic.

MAIDEN CEREMONY PHOTOS

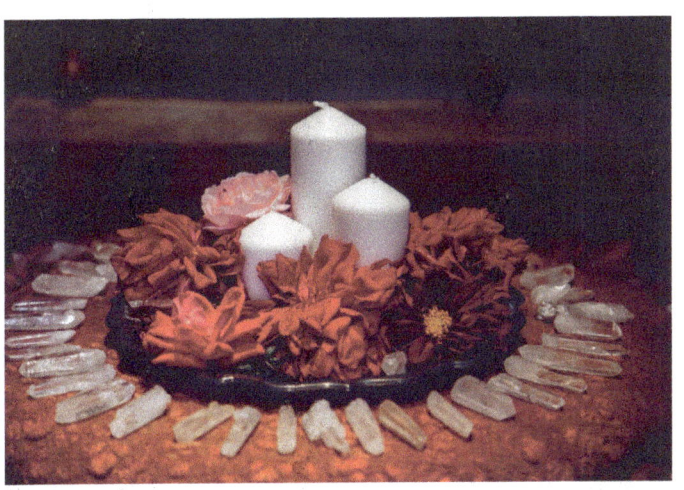

Central Altar with Maiden, Mother and Matriarch candles.

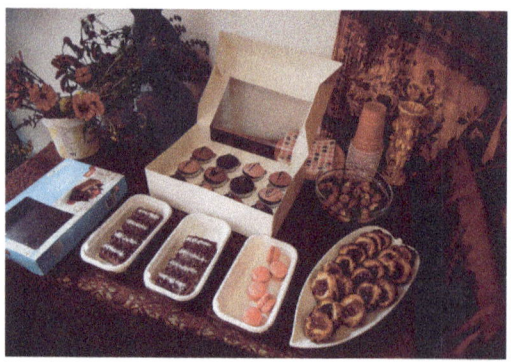

Delicious red treats.

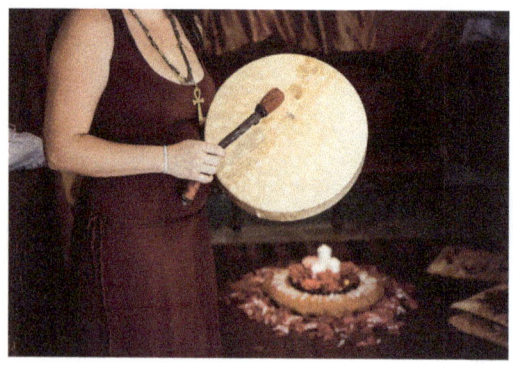

Drumming the primordial heartbeat of the Great Mother

MAIDEN CEREMONY PHOTOS | 93

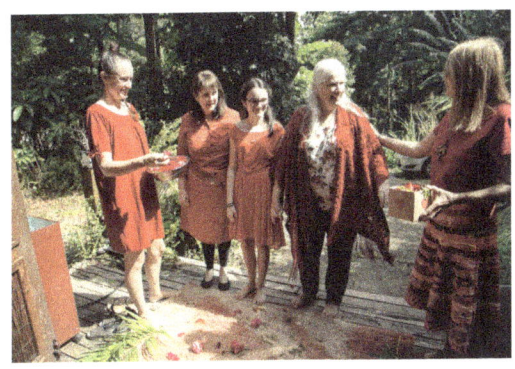

Grandmothers guiding Auraura (who was blindfolded beforehand) as Aunty Jo and Oma throw petals at her feet.

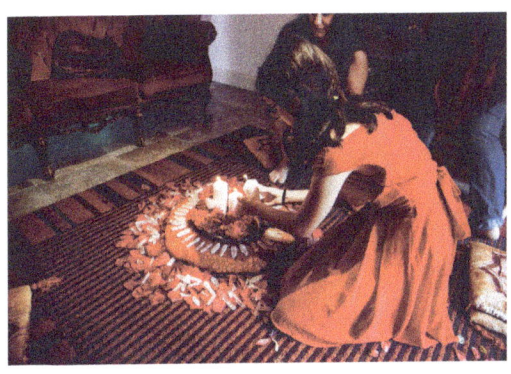

Auraura lighting her Maiden candle.

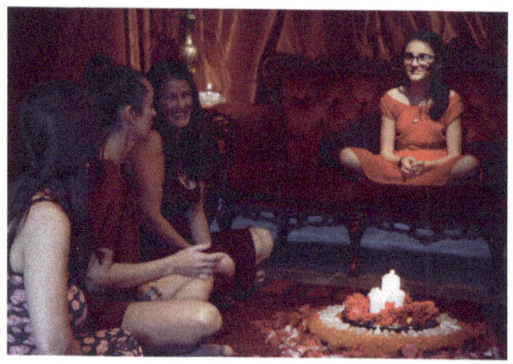

Sharing menarche and menstrual stories.

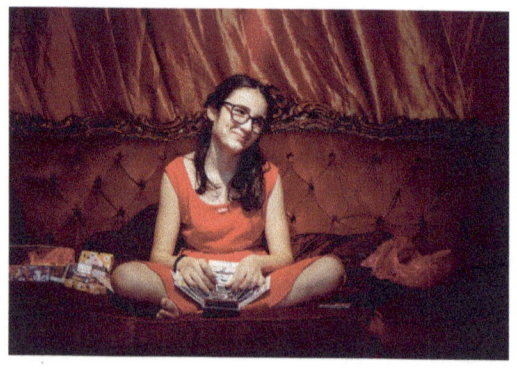

Receiving blessings and sentimental gifts.

MAIDEN CEREMONY PHOTOS | 95

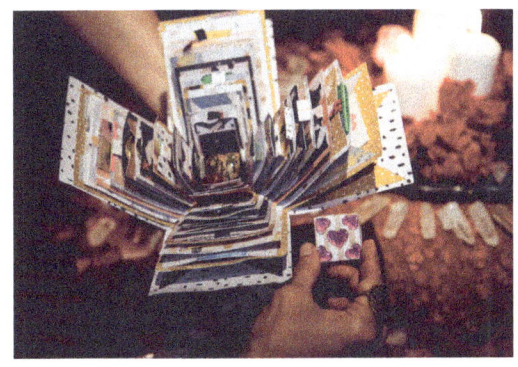

Auraura will always be NanaH's little Jelly Bean.

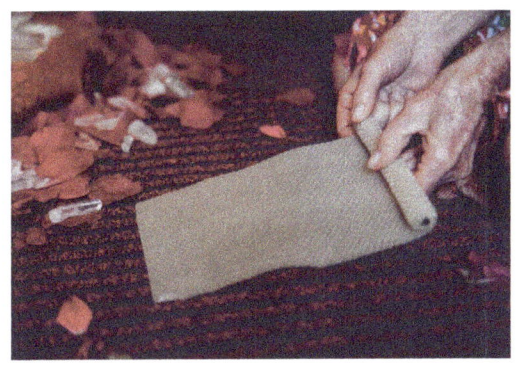

creating the rolled menstrual candle.

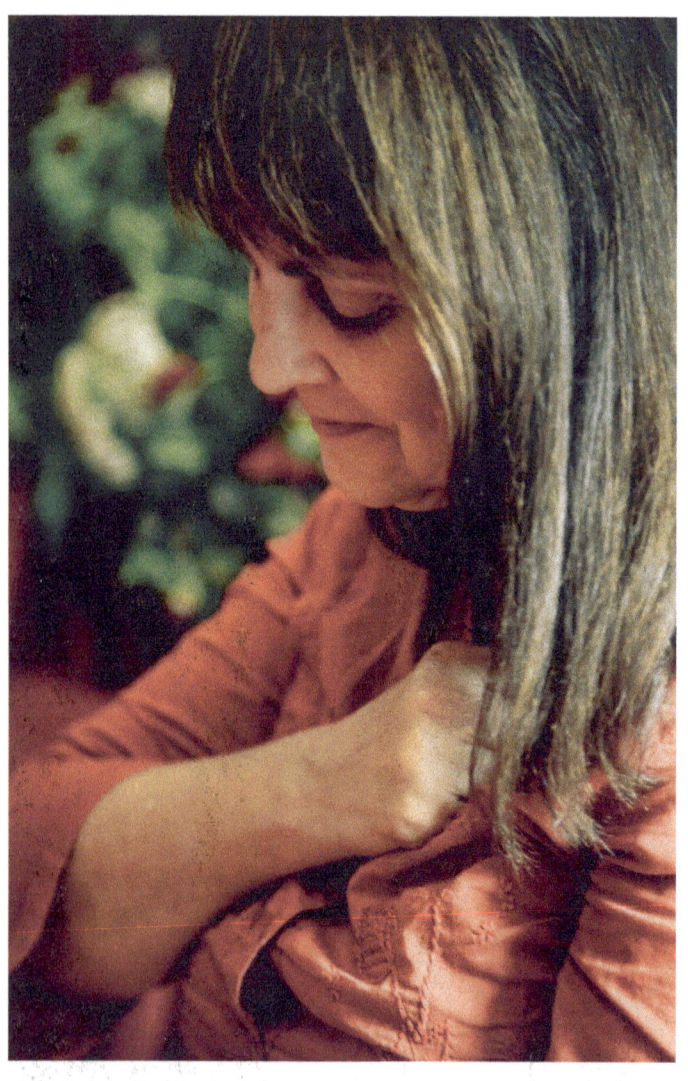

Ma, imbuing the special ankh pendant with her love and blessings.

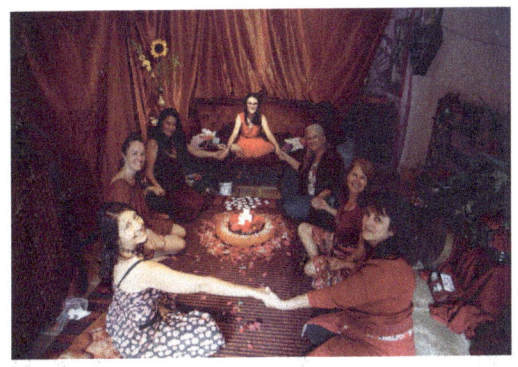

Closing Circle.

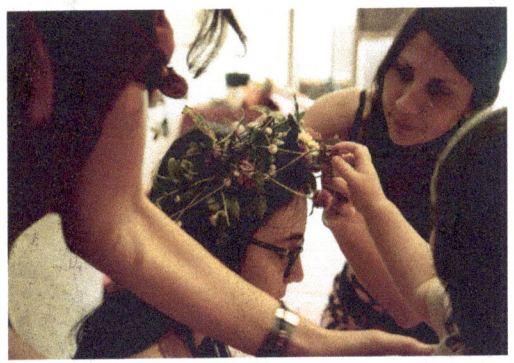

All hands on deck, Auraura being adorned with her flower-crown

98 | MAIDEN.

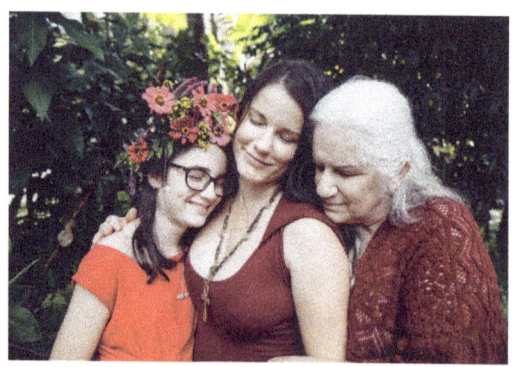

Triple Goddess Photoshoot.

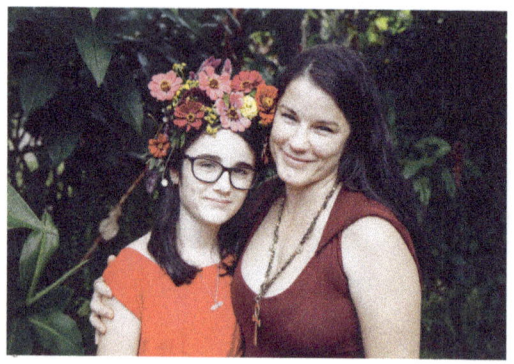

Maiden + Mother

6

HOW TO CREATE YOUR CEREMONY TEMPLATE

*I*f you are planning a ceremony that has a few elements to it, then you may like to come up with a template to help you weave each segment together in a harmonious and symbolic way. To create the 'bones' of the ceremony you will need some paper and a pen, and using the titles below, heart-storm and get your initial ideas down underneath, so that you can refine them into a "run-sheet" or script. This is an easy tool to follow, helping you stay focused on the actual day so you don't miss anything, which can happen if you are swept up in the moment. You can also use the Notes section in this book to jot down your ideas and prepare a draft.

OPENING-

Think of a powerful opening that is relevant to your event and sets the intention for your gathering together. This could be spoken intuitively in the moment, sharing a poem, song, drums, ringing a bell or healing bowl, sharing a story or quote, letters from loved ones, silence, cleansing ritual or cultural smoke/smudge tradition, etc. The whole idea is to create a moment that transitions everyone out of the everyday mundane into a ceremonial way of being present.

In my ceremonies I begin with inviting my guest to close their eyes and connect with their breath. I will then guide them to breathe deeply and will say something to the effect of:

> "I invite you now to take a deep breath, deep into the belly... relaxing the shoulders, relaxing the tongue, the jaw and brow. Bringing all of your awareness to the sensations in your body, the rhythm of your breath, the sounds in the room or outside. On your exhale I invite you to let out a gentle sound, a letting go... a deep sigh... letting go of any stories of the day, the journey here, the shuffling and juggling of roles and responsibilities to be here now, in this space and time."

<pause>

> "Before we begin ceremony today, I would first like to honour and acknowledge the traditional custodians of this land, the songlines and dreaming tracks of (State the original name of the custodians and Country you are on here). I would like to

honour and acknowledge my ancestors and your ancestors as we gather together to create a beautiful ceremony in honour and celebration of (Maiden's name) coming of age."

IT IS VERY important to make a conscious effort to acknowledge the traditional custodians of the land (by name if you can), your ancestors and guest's ancestors. This is a simple practice of respect and is worth the effort! This is often left out in many facilitator trainings, so be mindful of this and make the effort to know what country you are standing on! Obviously, if you a performing cultural ceremonies you would adhere to your traditional customs of doing things the proper way!

WELCOME-

How do you want to acknowledge and welcome your guests?

What important information do they need to know, like turning phones off, knowing where the toilets are, etc.?

What are your intentions for gathering?

INTRODUCTION-

Self explanatory- this is where the basic info for the ceremony is shared. Concepts, beliefs, the who, what, why and you can edify your guests as to what the process is and what to expect as well as sharing what boundaries are in place to keep it a safe and sacred space. This is especially important if personal stories are being shared.

One of the main ways that I do this is to give people a framework for contributing to the creation of a safe space by becoming a story keeper, which simply means, what happens in circle stays in circle. We do not gossip or discuss another person's story outside of the circle unless we have permission to do so.

TRANSITION-

How do you want to link to the next segment?

(Story sharing, quote/poem, song etc)

The transition is an uninterrupted flow from one activity to the next, like a segue.

RITUAL OR ACTIVITY-

This will be the part for a ritual ceremony- the part where the majick happens- the part of the most deepest significance- like the blessings + gift sharing part, the ritual candle making, red thread, etc. It's important to not have too many of these because it can be come quite overwhelming having so many activities. Keep it simple so these intimate moments are potent and powerful focal points of the whole ceremony. Choose which ones resonate from the previous chapter, or create your own!

(REPEAT THE TRANSITION/ RITUAL as many times as needed)

CLOSE-

What do you want to say that ends the event on a high note? What information is important for guests to know as you wrap it up? This is also a great opportunity to have a group photo whilst everyone is together in the moment.

PIECING IT ALL TOGETHER

Once you have your basic timeline you can now delve deeper into each section as to what happens during this specific time-frame, what is needed and how does it link or flow into the next segment.

A ceremony becomes Sacred and deeply meaningful because of the intricate and often subtle details which help to create an almost ethereal and otherworldly feeling.

You could type it up as if it were a play you were starring in with all the parts that you need to speak, aka your "lines", or you can create flash cards for the parts that you know you need to read from. It is totally up to you how you want to work; for the most part you want it to flow from you and through you as much as possible.

POTENT TRANSMISSIONS

Words are spells. There is so much power in not only what you speak, but more so HOW you speak. You don't need any acting skills to pull this off, what you need is PRESENCE!

HOW YOU SHOW UP is key!

Ceremony has the ability to transport you out of the mundane and into the mystical moment of the eternal now. Tone is everything. A great ceremonialist understands how to weave words that amplify the Spiritual energy of the moment in a way that suddenly, every word that is spoken becomes a sacred offering and prayer. Be mindful of the underlying cadence of your ceremonial script- it is important that it flows with grace, but also creates mood and tension when needed.

To make your words more potent, it is important to practice inflection and to know when to use a pause to create anticipation and evoke emotion. A great way to practice is to record yourself reading your script so you can get a feel for how you need to speak. You will notice a shift at some stage from your normal speaking voice into your ceremonial voice. It is often deeper and more rhythmic in execution. If you find your voice going into a higher pitch or the "head voice" it's usually an indication of nerves, or not truly believing what you are saying which is necessary to carry those deeper tones, as they come from embodied presence.

All in all, you need to be YOU and be present in your body, present with your beautiful daughter and any guests you are sharing this moment with.

Having a script or run sheet with you is a great way to make sure you don't forget anything and that the day flows effortlessly. If you find that you become nervous on the day, simply take a moment to come back to your breath, slow down and be present to the energy in the room. Sometimes, even with the most precise planning, things can go awry... if this arises I suggest you laugh it off and keep on keeping on. Trust in your ability to create something truly majickal and meaningful for your daughter and yourself. At the end of the day, you'll have a story to tell!

MENSTRUAL MAJICK AND THE CEREMONY OF BLEEDING

MYSTICAL WOMBSPACE

The Womb is a potent creative power centre. It is the original pristine portal of life as we know it, and we all know it.

This dark chasm is a Sacred portal, where we seed not only life but also ours (and others') dreaming, ideas and wisdom. We all start life in the dark container of *Wombman*, our first imprints are absorbed in the aquatic realms enveloped in Mother's sacred waters.

The *wombspace* is sacred, and as such is to be met with reverence and honour for it's innate wisdom and majick. The nature of the feminine expression is fullness... and so it becomes essential to tune into the womb centre to see what is stored there.

Just as a mermaid plunges the depths of the ocean in search for hidden treasures, one must dive deep into the internal realms to access and retrieve one's own innate wisdom.

WOMB WISDOM

The womb is a sacred container, a generator and incubator of creativity and intuition... a place to nurture life and dreaming. Because it is dark and energetically fertile with infinite creative potential, the womb becomes a great place to store and hide old emotions, tension and beliefs which become trapped and unable to flow or be released from the body in a somatic way. Just as we naturally shed from menses, we can also use the wisdom of the womb to release that which does not serve us, such as thoughts, emotions and subconscious beliefs and in doing so, realign to our creative potential- using the wombspace to grow and nurture our dreams and goals.

One of the easiest ways to heal and release whatever no longer serves is to work with the power of menstruation as a symbolic and visceral experience of letting go, of cleansing and releasing. This practice of tuning into the body, asking how you are feeling, what's not working, what emotions are stirring in the undercurrents, and then using the actual physical process of bleeding with the intention of releasing and healing is deeply personal and often cathartic. It makes the inner "shadow" work more real as you become actively engaged in mind, body and Soul.

Each day more women are realising that the menstrual cycle is not a burden but rather an amazing opportunity to journey deeper into the beauty and sacredness of being a woman. The womb is an untapped and unlimited resource of power and potential. During menstruation a woman is at the peak of her visionary and intuitive senses. When she allows the space to rest, she can open up to new worlds and begin to dream them into being, holding and incubating the visions in her wombspace, as if carrying the most precious child.

A woman's connection to her menstrual cycle is a sacred communion with the Divine, an ongoing intimate relationship between her and the Great Mother, Goddess, Spirit… SHE… whatever you want to call the divine intelligence that exists all around us. The metamorphic world of creation, of life, death and rebirth, exists here, in this experience. The womb is a place of remembering.

Menstruation is a process of transition, transformation and alchemy.

There is so much majick, power and wisdom available to women who are willing to lean in and listen to the womb as she speaks in many different ways. Sharing this wisdom with your daughter from the beginning will empower her throughout her reproductive years.

WOMB BLOOD IS SACRED

I came across Jasmin Starchild's work, Founder of the Red Moon Menstrual Medicine Movement, in 2008. It was one of those moments where information *synchromystically* lands in your lap, as if it's a gift you didn't know you needed at the time. I remember watching a youtube video where she said something to the effect of,

> "When women return their blood to the Earth, men will stop killing one another for what we can so easily offer".

This really resonated with me and it was the first time I began to connect with how Sacred my blood was. It was around this time that I received the inner wisdom that the blood should flow, and I stopped using tampons. I also experimented with free-bleeding and stepping out of the consumerist side of menstrual hygiene products and began to use cloth pads which I bought locally and still have to this day.

My vagina became a holy temple. Her blood was a sacrament to the Divine and my flow became an active ritual of life and death, in service to the great Mother of Creation. Up until my early 20's I was disconnected from the spiritual experience of my blood and so now I share this wisdom with my daughters.

I know that being 20 for some is considered early to be connected to menstruation as a spiritual experience, and I know this was only made possible by the amazing outspoken women who walked long before me and were bold enough to speak up and share their wisdom unashamedly even when it felt like no one was listening. We are listening now, more than ever before because we feel the deficit of these practices in our way of being and I believe there's a place deep inside of us that knows it is time for this collective wisdom to be shared. We must do this in a way that honours the legacy of these women who are now considered elders of this wisdom, some of which I have intentionally referenced in this book out of deep respect.

Over the years, I began to journey with my blood and started researching more about the power of the menstrual cycle because I knew there was a missing key to my journey as a woman. I knew there was something MORE to being cyclical. There were things that I was not taught. And this ancient, primal wisdom was being remembered by women all over the world, including myself!

This lead me to exploring the Women's Mysteries and the Red Tent Movement, and then onto creating the Kuranda Womb Temple and my Wise Wombman business and online Wisdom School.

I offered my blood back to the Earth in ritual. I tracked my cycle. I would anoint my third eye and heart with the first blood of the cycle and sit in quiet contemplation, tuning into my wombspace and inner worlds.

Connecting with my blood gave me a sense of returning home to my embodied wisdom and my inner power. I started having deeply symbolic and prophetic dreams. I started to trust my intuition and my womb as a compass to guide me in life. Even though sometimes the messages that I would receive from my inner oracle didn't make sense, I stayed true to honouring the choices that came to the surface from the deepest parts of me… My inner Wise Wombman.

She knows!

Working with Womb Blood is a beautiful Spiritual practice but it is also an important practice to notice any physical changes and variations in your blood colour and texture that may need to be addressed for health reasons. Womb blood should be healthy bright red at the beginning and end of the cycle, with a consistent flow that wanes to a light spotting. There should be no clots, dark colours or intense pain.

COLLECTING WOMB BLOOD

There are a few different ways your daughter can collect her blood that is safe and hygienic.

The womb sheds the lining at the end/beginning of our cycle, and the natural biological function is for this blood to flow out of the vagina. Common practice is to use disposable pads and tampons which not only absorb the flow of blood, but there are many nasty chemicals and bleaches connected with the processing of the cotton and they create so much waste that goes to landfill.

Natural, reusable alternatives that allow you to collect your womb blood are menstrual cups, made from surgical grade silicone, which sits inside the vagina close to the cervix and collects blood straight from the source. These are great to use if you are going to be practicing blood rituals and offering your blood back to the Earth.

Sponges and cloth pads are a natural alternative to cotton tampons and can be rinsed, cleaned and reused.

Menstrual pants allow the experience to free bleed whilst capturing menstrual blood in the fabric of the underpants.

These can all be soaked in water and wrung out to collect the blood to use in an offering.

MAJICKAL MOON CYCLES

A full lunar cycle as the moon moves through its different phases is 28 days. The average menstrual cycle of a woman is also 28 days. She too will move through different phases of her cycle, menstruation, the follicular phase, ovulation and the luteal phase.

Not all women are in sync with the moon, though a vast majority of women will find a correlation with their menstrual cycle and different phases of the moon. It is also interesting to note, that in times before electricity, many women's cycles would sync together around certain phases of the moon, and natural pregnancy would be timed with seasons that supported birth and the well-being of Mother and baby.

If you've ever live with women in the same house, it is likely that you will bleed together. How amazing is that!

Women who ovulate on the full moon and bleed on the new moon are connected to what is known as the White Moon Cycle, whereas women who ovulate with the new moon and bleed with the full moon are said to be in sync with the Red Moon Cycle. I learned this wisdom from Miranda Gray.

The White Moon cycle is the most common to sync with and calls women inwards. It is a time of inner journeywork, fertility, and personal growth.

The Red Moon is also a common cycle to sync with and calls women to their wisdom in service and leadership. It is a time of sharing yourself and holding space for others.

Both of these cycles work in symbiosis, when a Red Moon woman is menstruating she is held by the White Moon woman and vice versa. This provides a community approach to supporting each other with rest and renewal, emotional support and healing.

On either side of these are the transitional cycles that sync to the waxing and waning phases. The Waxing moon occurs after the New Moon and is symbolic of cultivating confidence in creativity, leaving the dark whilst regaining power and building strength. The Waning Moon occurs after the Full moon and is symbolic of the return to stillness and reconnecting to your inner wisdom and acknowledging what you've created.

It's also important to note that celestial events can affect the womb. Things such as super moons, blue moons and eclipses can all have an impact on the timing of the menstrual cycle and the intensity of experience, especially on an emotional level.

BLOOD RITUALS FOR TEENS

Offering womb blood back to the Earth directly is a powerful way to connect with Country and to cultivate a deep sense of place… of belonging and honouring. When one is connected to Country, one cares for it and preserves it for the future generations. The more we connect with the natural world, the more we begin to tap in to the language of place and we begin to walk gently with more connection and presence then ever before. Blood rituals do not need to be strange and witchy; they can be, if that's what you're into.

Blood rituals can be a simple and practical way to help your garden thrive, as well as a way to offer part of yourself, your DNA, to the landscape as way to interact with the intelligence that exists all around us. Life wants to create with us and through us. Working with menstrual blood may not be your cup of tea, and that is ok. I share this practical wisdom for those that feel the inherent majick and ceremony of bleeding.

If it resonates, teach your daughter how to collect her blood and offer it back to the Earth through ceremony, releasing anything that has not come to pass… any built up tension and emotion or expectations that she may be holding on to. On the last day of her bleed, she can gather the collected blood in a sacred chalice or vessel of some sort. Mixing with water to dilute, she can intone her offering with breath, prayers and gratitude. It is important that she find somewhere that she can offer the womb blood back in a relaxed and peaceful way. Encourage her to create a beautiful space, with flowers, crystals, candles and anything that is from the natural environment and evokes a sense of graceful beauty.

Remember, sometimes humble offerings can be exquisite in their simplicity. If you don't have access to natural environments, think about creating a balcony garden or feeding the indoor plants or perhaps she has a special one in a pot in her bedroom.

Gratitude is a great way to amplify manifestation abilities as it centres us in the heart. Energy flows where attention goes, so participating in Sacred rituals often, allows her to align her body, mind and spirit with her divine essence and power as a co-creator of this world. As she collects her blood, she can begin to feel the energy of gratitude swell inside and fill her wombspace. Focusing on the sensations in her body she then breathes it in, whilst handling her sacred womb blood. Intention and Presence is everything.

This is a ritual to shift the focus from all the woes of adolescence and intentionally release and let go of that which has not come to fruition that month, and to trust the greater weaving at play. As she offers the blood, she begins to visualise everything that is beautiful in her world. She may then like to use her creativity to express all that is good in her world.

It is beneficial that your daughter journal her experience during her sacred womb time. Having a book will help her create an inner dialogue so that she can deepen her understanding of how her mind works and to build emotional resilience.

Some journal prompts to share are as follows.

- *What are you feeling emotionally and in your body?*
- *What colour is your blood? - this is to monitor health and also if you are shedding the lining completely.*
- *Document what your flow is like- is it regular/heavy/spotting, etc.?*
- *What is happening in your personal life this month?*
- *What has come to fruition this month?*
- *What can you let go of?*
- *What are you still hoping to experience?*
- *What has been hard emotionally this month?*
- *Are you confused or anxious about anything?*
- *Are your relationships healthy?*
- *What shadow work have you experienced?*
- *What insights have you gathered this month, what have you learned about yourself?*
- *How have you nurtured yourself this month and how did it make you feel?*
- *What do you need right now?*
- *What are you grateful for?*
- *What is beautiful in your life right now?*

WOMB STEAMING

Womb Steaming is a beautiful and nourishing self-care ritual that supports us physically, emotionally and spiritually. Hydrotherapy has been used in many cultures around the world as is the practice of using steam and various different medicinal herbs to increase circulation to the pelvic organs. By using heat, which activates the healing properties of the essential oils in the plants released via the gentle steaming process, the womb steam can increase blood flow and circulation as well as balance hormones and treat infections and irregularities with the menstrual cycle. It is best to work under the guidance of a qualified practitioner. I have been working with Venus V-Steam herbals for a few years with great results.

You can work with organic dried herbs, or pick them fresh from your garden. Mugwort is a great all rounder, as well as tulsi, motherwort, chamomile, hibiscus and rose. Most aromatic herbs are great to use, although you may want to work with specific plant medicines to treat any irregularities, in this case it is wise to work closely with a qualified practitioner who knows the properties of the plants and can create a steaming protocol to work with them safely. Never use essential oils undiluted from a bottle. These are too potent and can cause irritation and burning.

The ratio for usage is usually a cup of herbs to around 2 litres of water in pot. Bring this to the boil slowly and make sure you leave the lid on. Take the pot off the heat and place it in position. You can use an old commode, a custom steaming stool, an upcycled chair with a hole cut out. Whatever you use, make sure it is a natural, unvarnished material. Place pillows under your feet to keep your knees slightly higher than your hips and pelvis. You can even squat over the pot, but that's not very comfortable for long sessions. Depending on the season, you may like to drape blankets around yourself to keep the warmth in. Steaming can be done in many different variations from 5-30 minutes. If at any time you feel that it is too hot, adjust your position so as to avoid a steam burn or overheating.

Inviting your daughter to try womb steaming can be very beneficial to her holistic womb care, especially during a time where her hormones are in such rapid changes from puberty. It's also a great opportunity to soften into stillness, to listen to beautiful music or journal. Creating space for "me" time as she will come to know and love it.

THE RED TENT MOVEMENT.

Coined from Anita Diamant's book of the same name, The Red Tent is a sacred place where women come together in solidarity for connection, healing, creativity, storytelling, education and empowerment. Although menstrual huts are documented in many indigenous tribes and in some areas still used today, The Red Tent is a modern adaptation in that women gather in a safe communal place, usually decorated with red textiles symbolic for the blood we shed as women, to share stories and wisdom. Currently there is a global movement and revival of these much-needed spaces and sacred women's circles.

In 2012, Isadora Liedenfrost's documentary, *"Things We Don't Talk About, women's stories from the Red Tent"* captured a beautiful blueprint of what these modern spaces can look and feel like. The film shares wisdom from many world renowned leaders including the noteworthy pioneers, Alisa Starkweather from the Red Tent Temple Movement and DeAnna L'am from the Red Moon School of Empowerment and Red Tent's in Every Neighbourhood, both of which have been creating women's empowerment spaces for decades. The film invites you to experience what the Red Tent can look and feel like in different communities, where the common thread that is woven through all of them is a sense of safety for women to rest and share their stories, connect with other women and heal their trauma. Young women are welcomed into the Red Tent and offered wisdom from their elders to help them understand their bodies, fertility, the initiations into different seasons of womanhood and tools to navigate life as a woman in the modern world.

I have been creating and facilitating women's circles for over a decade now, with the birth of the Kuranda Womb Temple and now a scaled back version, which is a monthly gathering called the Cairns Sacred Women's Circle. Women and young girls are welcomed into this space, and I am so grateful that my daughters have access to this as a "normal" part of life that supports their mental, emotional and spiritual health and wellbeing. They have witnessed the majick of connection; solidarity and sisterhood as I would call the women in to a circle setting to share stories, to laugh, sing, dance, play and heal. I have witnessed incredible transformations in women's lives who have journeyed with me over the years, most of whom felt like their body and nervous system had a chance to settle in these safe spaces, as if they felt a welcoming and deep remembering take place. A common story was that many women didn't know they needed circle, until they found it.

Women need access to these types of spaces, whether it is a place completely decorated with red fabrics and cushions, outside in nature or shared cups of tea over the dining room table. We need safe places to drop the masks we adopt and the characters we play in life, to return to a place of authenticity and sovereignty. As a mentor and educator I have been training women how to create and facilitate these safe spaces so that they can serve their communities in a way that nourishes the heart and soul of their participants, because what works for one, does not always work for all and so the key is to honour diversity in a way that brings forth connection. The more women who feel the calling of this service work and step forward to honour it, the more diversity we have which creates healthy communities, locally and globally.

In the past couple of years I have noticed a new wave of circles being birthed in that they are dedicated to our young girls and teens. These young girls or maiden circles are an initiation into creating and upholding the codes of sisterhood, upholding values of connection, kindness, healthy relationships and empowerment. Some of these circles provide young girls with the education to prepare for menstruation, whilst others focus on imprinting strong foundations of self-esteem and body positivity to create resilience as our youth face incredible challenges in this technocratic world. I find that this is the next phase of service work, for young girls to feel that sense of belonging and kinship as they gradually move through the processes of initiation into the depths of the women's mysteries.

FINAL WORDS OF WISDOM

Puberty is a Sacred Rite of Passage. It can be a lonely and confusing time where young girls are imprinting powerful beliefs around what it means to be a woman.

As a mother, the greatest work we can do is in rearing children who are healthy (in mind, body and Spirit), grounded and connected to the world in a way that naturally encourages them to share of themselves in genuine, creative and courageous ways.

As a Matriarch you have the power to create an incredible legacy that lives through and beyond you, for you can never truly comprehend the vast reach of the ripples this work creates.

All in all, initiating your daughter into deep embodiment practices is going to require you to lead by example. Monkey see, monkey do, so to speak.

The reason why I have included all of this in the book is because I know that for some, seeing puberty, menarche and maidenhood as something Sacred, is all new. And that is ok. You may not have had the type of initiations presented in this book, but when you know better, you do better. So if this is new, what a beautiful and powerful way to connect and bond with your blossoming daughter as you both learn and grow together.

There is always time to connect and heal.

The bond between mother and daughter is so special, and I hope that this guidebook has provided you the wisdom, humour and resources necessary for you to initiate your daughter in a potent and deeply meaningful way. Majick is available to those who seek it.

There is a change happening collectively.
Peace on Earth begins with birth.

The birth of Babies.
The birth of Maidens.
The birth of Mothers

… The birth of Wisdom Keepers.

Wherever you are on your journey, whatever season you are in… You are powerful, you are beautiful and what you do matters. This work sends powerful ripples into the future, helping women return to their inner wisdom and power. Please share what you have learned with women in your community. Together we can shift the paradigm of shame in one generation. Liberation comes from education and sharing of wisdom to help heal the whole.

Thank you for reading. So much love and many blessings to you and your family.

Remember to access the wisdom within.

Donna Raymond xx

AURAURA'S EXPERIENCE- IN HER WORDS

MY MENARCHE STORY

The earliest memories I have of mum showing and explaining what moon cycles were, was when I was like three or something when mum called me from down the hallway. I came running down, in my little cute purple skirt. Mum was explaining to me what periods are. Other times it was mum showing me how to put a pad on. Each year, she would explain it to me with more depth and I got more and more excited to get my own. It's hard for me to explain what it was like because it's completely normal for me and it's nothing out of the ordinary. At home when I have a question, I'm not embarrassed by talking about it, even if it's in front of the guys in my family. I was raised to know that our cycles are natural and shameless. Mum also taught me what to expect, as I grew older. When my bleed did come I wasn't nervous, instinctively I knew exactly what to do, it didn't surprise me.

The morning after I got my menarche, I got to skip

school, and mum took me to my favourite café to celebrate. It was amazing, I felt different, but I also felt myself. It was a weird experience, but I felt very overwhelmed and happy, it was just all mixed emotions.

That afternoon, Mum drove me to the river. She told me to find a place to sit, whilst she waited back a little to get something for me. Eventually she came over and put her arms around me close and tight and told me to close my eyes. We walked closer to the water, she sat me down on a comfy mat, I could hear the water rushing against the sand, the wind and rustling of paper. I opened my eyes, to see a basket layered with pink tissue paper and a fresh bunch of flowers. Inside was a card, a box of pads, liners, a big pouch (inside were reusable cloth pads), a box of Ferrero Rochers (my favourite) and a bottle of clary calm essential oil. This was so exciting! It was like a big period care package. I think the best part was the flowers (I love flowers!)

After eating two chocolates (LOL) we laid down and talked about menarche related stuff in such a humorous way that I wasn't afraid to ask weird questions.

I knew mum was planning a special ceremony for me because she asked for my permission, which I agreed to. I requested not to be told about anything as I only get one menarche ceremony in my life… right! We joked about having yoni cakes we thought it would be hilarious. The night before the ceremony I was staying at my dad's house. All I was told was to wear a red dress and to get my beauty sleep and to be prepared for the next day. When I arrived back home, I wasn't allowed to go through the front because that's where the ceremony space was set up. I didn't know what to expect, as my mother isn't predictable.

I remember my two loving grandmothers, leading me

into the ceremony. I could see my aunty and my step-grandmother throwing flowers at my feet whilst my mother and my stepmother drummed on their homemade skin drums. When I sat down on the red velvet couch I felt so special and happy. To start the ceremony, my mum, my grandmother and I all lit a candle each and placed them on the central altar. Everyone all shared the stories of their first bleed. Some were really upsetting and some were full of laughter, which brought humour to the circle. It was at that moment that I felt like I was a part of something bigger or as though I was in a secret club.

It surprised me how little I knew about the women in my family when it comes to their menarche especially my grandmothers. They spoke about how it was so hard and well… different in their time.

Overall the ceremony was what I expected it to be and more. We ate yoni cupcakes, we laughed, we cried, I got beautiful gifts that I will treasure forever. All the beautiful women in my life made me a flower crown and we also had a photoshoot at the end. I believe that day was the most joyful memorable day ever!!! Later that night my mum, my nanaH and I had a private ritual in the back yard.

Since then I have been using the journal that mum gave me by tracking my cycle and learning the pattern of my emotions and my mood. It surprises me so much that when I'm about to bleed I find myself being more introverted than my normal self, I also find my self arguing with my dad about how I'm not being anti-social (but all I want is to be by myself lol!)

Lately I feel as though I am more myself and welcomed more to be a maiden.

My wish is that all girls should be welcomed into maidenhood by being celebrated, instead of being embarrassed and ashamed of it.

Auraura Freedom

-over and out-
October 2020

WORDS FROM NANAH

An invitation to my eldest granddaughters Mense Celebration is something that I will never forget. I listened to the stories of the significant women in her life as they shared the memory of their first bleed. We honoured her, talking and laughing and shedding tears together, breaking the cycle of shame replacing it with a celebration, embracing and nurturing the changes that come with the flow of first blood.

As women we know it is the most purest of pure, connecting us to not only other women but our ancestors, Mother Nature, and the universe. It is in essence a life form, it is bleeding women who allow humankind to exist. That's something that should be celebrated not shunned upon.

We were to bring a gift for Auraura to acknowledge her transition from child to maiden and after much thought I knew exactly what my gift would be. Since her birth I had always called her "Jelly Bean" so I knew my gift had to reflect that. I created an explosion box embellished with photo memories of her life thus far.

Auraura took time reminiscing over the photos smiling, sometimes with embarrassment but nevertheless I could see her emotions taking over. I encouraged her to keep going as there were 13 boxes one for each year of her human existence and at the rate she was going it was going to take a long time to get to the final box. Finally she opened the last little box about a centimetre square in size. Auraura looked at me and eye to eye the tears welled up as the significance of the small **RED JELLY BEAN** that was resting safely inside this small box triggered the connection we had with each other. I could see she was overwhelmed as was I and tears of love flowed from us both.

My menarche story, well it was 1972, I was 17 and any matters relating to puberty or sex education were not discussed in my family. Menstruation was like the plague had to be kept very hush hush. I would hear the girls talk of the "time of the month" or "their friend had come to visit". All my friends had started their periods long before me. I did wonder when my time would come, but my main focus was fitting in with the other girls in my school class. Flat chested me had not even earned the privilege of wearing a bra, nor did I really want to. I woke to find a rusty colour goop in my knickers, it took a moment to realise, holy shit I've got my period! I was not sure what to do, it was a school day and I had to do something quickly, so it was off with the undies! I wrapped them in another pair and put them into my top drawer to be dealt with when I got home from school, trusting and praying my mother would not find them.

Now what?!

(*Light bulb moment* I Invade my older sisters drawers.)
Yep "Modess" pads and a sanitary belt!

Let me explain… It was an actual elastic belt used to hold sanitary pads in place. Basically just an elastic loop that goes around your hips, with small clips hanging in the front and back, which you then attached a sanitary pad to. It took a bit to work out the fitting of pad to the belt. I knew this piece of elastic and I were not going to have a long acquaintance. I was too scared, yes scared to tell Mum…so my piece of elastic and I went to school. I could hear the other girls whispering as I had been the only girl who hadn't "started". I was so embarrassed. I knew it was about the way I was walking. The worst thing was that the elastic belt would twist and dig into my skin. I could not wait till end of day when a visit to the chemist was inevitable.

Tampons or stick on pads?

Ads on TV about tampons depicting what a revolutionary invention they were allowing the wearer to ride horses and even swim with them. OK tampon it is! Not sure what I should get I just picked up the first packet I saw on the shelf, TAMPAX I remember the brand vividly. What came next was a lesson well learnt. Not bothering to read the instructions I did not realise that you had to remove the cardboard applicator. So you can imagine or maybe not how insanely, uncomfortable these things were. It wasn't until I did read the instructions I learnt I had shoved a telescope like piece of cardboard into my pubescent 'what's e me call it', no wonder it was painful! Ok so this brand was not working for me. Off to the chemist again to purchase the advertised revolutionary brand on TV – Carefree Tampons.

Back at home sitting on the loo carefully reading instructions so as not to make another mistake, I looked at all the diagrams and positioned myself exactly how the instructions suggested. It felt like I was a dog cocking his leg to pee. But here goes uhhhhh that's arrrr inserted. Phew. At least walking was much easier and actually couldn't really feel anything. Except this piece of string that had found its way to a place that was not very comfortable. After a little bit of manoeuvring I was confident I had mastered the tampon insertion. Back at home I still had to address the bloody knickers. So my knickers had a bath with me that night. I washed and washed even used the scrubbing bush but no amount of washing was working, my knickers were still stained. Paranoid my mother would find out I disposed of them in the trash wrapped up in and empty cereal box.

Lessons learnt from my first period. 1 Read instructions carefully. Something I now do with any new purchases. 2 Blood stains – soak in cold water immediately to avoid permanent staining. In conclusion I know my mother did not take the time to educate me in the whole process of becoming a woman and in her defence not sure I did either with my daughters. However I am so gratefully that my grand daughter was honoured in a way she will treasure always. Thank you to her Mother for making that possible.

- Heather Raymond
    aka Mum and NanaH
    Jan 2021

FIND A WOMEN'S CIRCLE

In 2014 ***The Divine Feminine App*** was created by Caryn MacGrandle and is the world's largest listing of women's circles and events. I was fortunate enough to watch this project come to fruition and support it during its early days. It is a fantastic platform to locate or list an event in your community.

- **Caryn MacGrandle: thedivinefeminineapp.com**

Having said that, I have also listed facilitators and communities below, so please reach out to those in your area and if you want to learn how to become a confident leader of this type of work there are many educators around the world who you can learn from, in person and online, myself included. *Sacred Circle Secrets* is one of my signature home study programs and also the foundational facilitator training for my Wisdom Keeper Initiates, which is a 1on1 mentorship program. I also offer training on Sacred Ceremony and personalised mentorship programs.

AUSTRALIA

Cairns

Donna Raymond, Wise Wombman

Sacred women's circles, Sacred Rites of Passage events and ceremonies, facilitator training and business mentoring.

-www.donnaraymond.com.au

- www.wisewombman.com

Kim Darby

the Yaya Sisterhood Empowerment circles for girls 8-12 and first moon circles.

- www.sisterrisecollective.com.au

@sisterrisecollective

Kathy Popplewell

Daintree Love

www.kathypopplewell.com

Ashley Thrives

Divinely Woman, Women's Circles and Sacred Rites of Passage Ceremonies

www.divinelywoman.com

Jillian Zamora-

Womens Retreats, drum circles and Rites of Passage Ceremonies

—

www.zamama.love

www.rewilding.love

@zamamashamana

Jassie Maude, Womens Circles+ Womb Healing

www.facebook.com/Jassie.Maude

QUEENSLAND-

Marissa Reid, Magnetic Island

A Soulful Journey with Marissa Reid. Energy Healings, Women's Circles, Holistic Counselling

www.marissareid85.wixsite.com/asoulfuljourney

marissareid85@gmail.com

Marie Zonruiter, Yeppoon

Women's Circle and Maidenhood Ceremonies
www.bondoulahealings.com.au

https://www.facebook.com/BondoulaHealings

Kiera Douglas, Sunshine Coast

Women's and Teen circles, Rites of Passage transitions

Instagram @_Sacredspaces

Kiera.douglas04@gmail.com

Shekinah Leigh, Gold Coast

Coming of age programs for 9-13year old and Mother and daughter events

https://shekinahleigh.com.au/shakti-circles/

Rowena Hobbins, Gold Coast

Sacred Women's Circles and full moon circles for women and girls.

www.raisingup.com.au

https://www.facebook.com/raisingupwithrowena

https://www.instagram.com/raising_up_

hello@raisingup.com.au

NSW

Charlotte Pointeaux, NSW Southern Highlands

First Moon (Menarche) circles for girls aged 9-12 with their mothers. Monthly girls moon circles and First Moon Facilitator training.

charlotte@charlottepointeaux.com

-www.firstmooncircles.com

www.Instagram.com/first_moon_circles

Kitty Taylor-Ginesi, Picton NSW

facebook.com/Yogawithcatwollondilly

Adrienne Rhoads, Port Macquarie

First Moon Circles and friend group circles.

Contact: adriennerhoads@gmail.com

VICTORIA

Bek Grundy
Sacred Women's Circles

bekahbutterfly@gmail.com (Geelong)

SOUTH AUSTRALIA

Silvana Vagnoni, Adelaide

Womens Retreats and SHE CONNECTS gathering

-www.silvanavagnoni.com

Lora Love, Willunga, S.A

Reservoir of Rhythms, Maidens drum and voice circle. Circles and playshops for women of all ages

www.facebook.com/reservoirofrhythms

Instagram.com/reservoir_of_rhythms

Artemis WS House, Aldgate Adelaide Hills

Celebration day for girls, empowerment preparation for 10-12yr old girls and their mother's before menarche.

www.she-awakening.com.au

Instagram.com/she_awakening

WESTERN AUSTRALIA

Sophie Wicksteed, Perth

Sacred Women's Circles, Rites of Passage Ceremonies

https://www.facebook.com/theredyurt/

Michelle Coppard, Perth

Sacred Women's Circles

michelle.coppard@gmail.com

TASMANIA

Sharon Woolley Newstead, Tasmania.

First Moon For Girls Facilitator, Menstrual Cycle Coach, Natural fertility specialist -

www.sharonwoolley.com.au

NEW ZEALAND

http://www.tuitrust.org.nz/events/calendar/

EUROPE

Anne-Marie Owen, Somerset, UK

Sacred Women's Circles (Celtic traditions)

www.dunalife.org.

Nisha Toppin, Devon, UK

Period Health Matters

1-1 Period Health Coaching, Online First Moon Circles for pre teen girls & their mothers/ female carers, Celebration Day for Girls workshops, Menarche Gift Boxes, Women's Circles.

www.periodhealthmatters.com

@periodhealthmatters

nisha@periodhealthmatters.com

Katinka Soetens

pathoflovemysteryschool.com

www.Goddessconference.com

Corinna Didjurgeit, (Germany)

Young women Rite of Passage Ceremonies and programs

www.CorinnaDidjurgeit.com

Elise Petit, France

www.elisepetit.fr

Lunna Valerie Pergay , Paris

Red tent and rites of passage

www.facebook.com/valerie.pergay

Rose Caruana, Malta

Sacred Women's Circles and Ceremonies

www.facebook.com/rose.benito.56

Adriana Vais, County Sligo, Ireland

Women's and Maiden's circles

www.avwitchshop.com

instagram.com/adrianna_avwitchshop

USA

Asheville red tent movement

Ali M. Schaffer, Indianapolis, IN.

Shamanic Priestess & Naturopath - Your Tribe Sacred Circles, Red Tent Indy, Whole Holistic Soul Centre.

wholesoulcentre@gmail.com

redtentindy@gmail.com,

divinetribe7@gmail.com

Graell Corsini, Ashland

Goddess Temple of Ashland.

www.goddesstempleashland.com/

Aurora Rae FaeTerra

Red Tent and Women's Circles

https://faeterra.com/redtent/

Kelsey McEuen, South Oregon
Coming of age ceremonies for Maidens
www.wildmoondoula.com
instagram.com/wildmoon_doula

Jennifer Joy- "Magical Maidens"
https://magical-mama.com

Angel Aquarian, Big Island, Hawaii
Women's Circles and Menstrual Wisdom
Honoringthesacredself@gmail.com
instagram.com/theislandangel

ABOUT THE AUTHOR

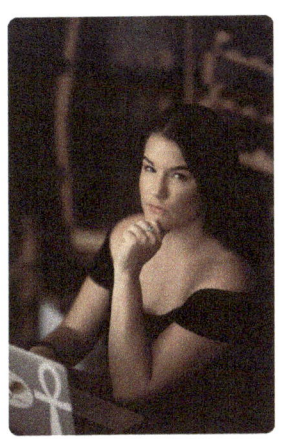

Donna Raymond is a humble visionary, ceremonialist, mentor and mother of 4 residing in the quaint rainforest village of Kuranda in North Queensland, Australia. Over the last decade she has created hundreds of women's circles, workshops, ceremonies, transformational healing journeys and offers online learning, training and menoring through her **Wise Wombman Wisdom School** which serves as a platform to educate, empower and inspire change in the world.

Connect with Donna Raymond www.WiseWombman.com
www.DonnaRaymond.com.au
Facebook: @wisewombmandreaming
Instagram: @wise_wombman
YouTube: ConsciousD

WISE WOMBMAN WISDOM SCHOOL

A portal for Sacred Feminine Wisdom, Soulful Leadership and Self Empowerment for Women, Modern Mystics and Visionary Creatives.

In a time of dramatic change, overwhelming sensory experiences, emotional instability and a seeming lack of intimacy and depth in the lives of many, Wise Wombman serves as a Modern Mystery School that strives to bring connection and meaning back into the lives of women and men around the world.

Conceived and created by Donna Raymond, Wise Wombman is an education platform dedicated to exploring and sharing Sacred Feminine Wisdom that is deeply spiritual and practical in application.

Wise Wombman is a conduit and catalyst for catharsis and personal transformation, facilitating healing and inner journeywork to encourage and support others as Sovereign beings, co-creators, respectful community-minded individuals and powerful wisdom keepers.

Online courses and journey work through the inner realms of the psyche and womb space have been mapped and delivered in such a way, so as to spark a sense of remembering, allowing pathways to come back to Self beyond story, trauma and ancestral imprints, initiating one into a space of liberation, emotional resilience, self-empowerment and leadership.

DOWNLOAD YOUR FREE MAIDEN MENSTRUAL CALENDAR

https://www.wisewombman.com/maiden-menstrual-calendar/

RELEVANT OFFERINGS

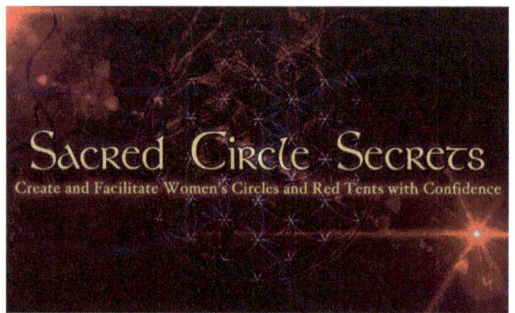

Sacred Circle Secrets is a self guided, transformational training program designed to take all the pressure and stress out of learning to become a facilitator of Sacred Women's Circles, so that you can create and hold your own events with confidence and ease.

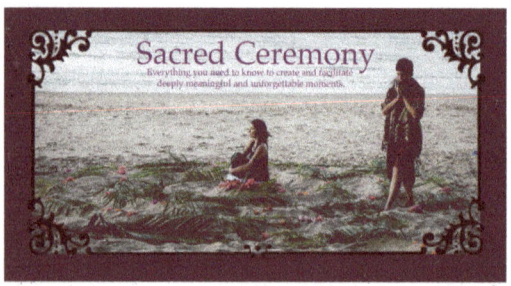

Sacred Ceremony- Everything you need to know to become a respectful and deeply embodied Ceremonialist that is capable of creating and facilitating Sacred Ceremonies including Rites of Passage.

NOTES...

www.ingramcontent.com/pod-product-compliance
Lightning Source LLC
Chambersburg PA
CBHW062038290426
44109CB00026B/2657